ENERGETIC EATING

LIVE BOLDLY BEYOND DIETING

BY HELEN BIRNEY, M.ED., INHC

Energetic Eating

Copyright © 2025 Helen Birney

All rights reserved. No part of this publication may be reproduced, distributed, or transmitted in any form or by any electronic or mechanical means, including photocopying, recording, or information storage and retrieval systems, without prior written permission in writing of Thought Leader Academy Publishing, or its duly authorized agent, except in the case of brief quotations embodied in reviews and certain other non-commercial uses permitted by copyright law. For information regarding permission, contact the publisher.

Cover design by Claudine Mansour Design. Interior design by Michael Beas.

Paperback ISBN: 979-8-9922573-5-9

Disclaimer: The following is for informational and entertainment purposes only and should not be considered financial or health advice. Readers are responsible for their mental and physical health and choices. Always consult with a financial advisor and mental health professional before making important decisions. Some names and distinguishing characteristics of individuals and organizations represented in this book have been changed to respect confidentiality. While best efforts have been made in preparing this book, the author and publisher make no warranty, representation, or guarantee with respect to the accuracy or completeness of information contained herein.

Published by Thought Leader Academy Publishing
3901 North Kildare Ave
Chicago, IL | 60641

To my daughters–
You are my "why." You gave me the strength to transform my struggles into purpose.

TABLE OF CONTENTS

Author's Note — 1

Introduction — 4

PART I: THE ENERGETIC EATING METHOD — 13

Chapter 1
The Five Commitments — 14

Chapter 2
The Triad of Health — 22

Chapter 3
Your Best Energetic Self — 26

PART II: THE SIX PILLARS OF ENERGETIC EATING — 37

Chapter 4
Pillar 1: Your Thoughts — 38

Chapter 5
Pillar 2: Your Mood — 72

Chapter 6
Pillar 3: Your Digestion — 109

Chapter 7
Pillar 4: Your Focus — 146

Chapter 8
Pillar 5: Your Energy Levels — 175

Chapter 9
Pillar 6: Conscious Choices   204

PART III: BRINGING IT ALL TOGETHER   229

Chapter 10
Prioritizing Your Health Brings Joy and Balance   230

Chapter 11
Looking Back, Looking Forward   241

Chapter 12
Energetic Eating Method Client Success Stories   248

Acknowledgments   259

About the Author   261

AUTHOR'S NOTE

Writing *Energetic Eating* has been a deeply personal and transformative journey. This book is for every woman who has ever felt stuck in a cycle of diets, self-doubt, and the frustration of not seeing the results she deserves. I understand because I've been there too. I've wrestled with the same questions: What am I missing? Why does lasting change feel so hard?

Through my own journey and years of coaching, I've learned that health is never one-size-fits-all. I spent over two decades caught in cycles of weight gain and loss, struggling to trust my body. Your path may look different, but the truth remains: health isn't just about what's on your plate or the number on the scale. It's about aligning with your goals, honoring your body, and choosing self-love every step of the way.

As you move through this book, you'll notice its progression—from dropping the diet narrative to a deeper exploration of whole-body health. This structure mirrors my journey and the one I hope to guide you on. First, we let go of restrictive mindsets and unsustainable approaches. Then, we learn how to listen to our bodies and celebrate our inherent worth.

To enhance your experience with *Energetic Eating*, I've created a dedicated book portal with resources, downloads, and additional tools to support you on your journey. Simply scan the QR code included throughout this book.

To living boldly beyond dieting,
Helen

Always consult your primary care physician before discontinuing the use of prescription medications or beginning any new health program. The recommendations from this book are not meant to diagnose, treat, or cure medical conditions, illness, and/or disease. The reader expressly assumes the risks inherent in making any psychological, nutritional, or lifestyle changes.

INTRODUCTION

I have been through countless diets to manage my weight: counting points, counting calories, counting macros, a random Chinese herb I found online, my made-up rainbow diet, juice fasts, cleanses, fat-based, plant-based, clean eating, intermittent fasting, and more. I believed that if I found the right diet and I could put my mind to it, I would stop gaining weight over and over again. But all it led me to was feelings of frustration with my body and shame on the scale. I stepped on scales countless times over twenty years—in my house, at weight-loss groups, at friends' and strangers' homes, rest stops, gyms, and hotels.

Now, I won't say you can't want weight loss—you can. There are practical health and confidence reasons that drive a desire to lose weight. But in my experience, when it takes center stage, that desire gets in the way of how you live your life. You hide in family pictures, make up excuses to miss important events, dedicate yourself to diets and exercise that keep you from enjoying time with friends and family, avoid wearing bathing suits, waste mental space thinking about your body when you look in the mirror, and adjust the way you sit or stand or hold your arms. Out of self-blame, self-criticism, and fear of constantly feeling this way, women turn to diets to fix themselves with a set of rules instead of *listening* to what their bodies need.

I thought weight loss was the answer to loving my body, and I thought a diet plan was how I would get there. But after one pivotal moment, I finally realized my decades-long struggle wouldn't go away until I broke free of the emotional bondage of choosing weight loss over loving myself, again and again and again.

It was early 2018. I didn't know it at the time, but it would be the last diet I'd ever try—30 days of eating only fruits, vegetables, and animal protein, as well as app tracking, calorie counting, fat-bomb coffees, and intermittent fasting.

I decided this "Frankendiet" would be the key—all the latest dieting trends I knew at the time blended into one. I really believed my body would finally lose weight and be free from ever longing for the number on the scale.

But what happened to me was the opposite of freedom.

Every night, during my 30-day "Frankendiet" plan, I went to bed with horrible chest pain. It would start under my ribs, radiate around my heart, and take my breath away. I'd wake up throughout the night, sweating through my sheets, terrified I was having a heart attack.

I dismissed the possibility that there was a problem with what I was doing. I wanted to prove that my efforts would release the next 10 pounds on the scale. I wanted to be the weight I always dreamed I could be. I wanted to mirror the confidence I saw on social media (#bodygoals!)—in fresh-faced women with tiny waists and magazine-ready images. So I kept going for weeks, ignoring messages from my body that this wasn't right and, more importantly, wasn't *safe* for me.

My best friend and I were dieting together, and the two of us, with the greatest intentions (and often joking about our future "bikini bodies"), supported each other on our weight-loss journeys. This wasn't our first 30-day diet commitment. Five years earlier, when we were raising our baby girls together and wanted to shed the post-partum weight, she shared a 30-day plan with me, which promised to be a new way of eating that would bring about more energy, less bloating, and weight loss. Early on, it didn't disappoint; I experienced many of those things. I got the itch to try it whenever I would put the weight back on, over and over again.

But every time I tried a 30-day program after that first effort, I failed. I desperately wanted the same results. I was chasing the rush I felt when I had precise control over my food intake and the exhilaration I felt when I put on a slim pair of jeans and a backless shirt without worrying about the parts of my body I hated.

So, here we were again. Five years and many failed attempts later, making the same 30-day commitments, expecting the same drastic results. We took turns stepping on the scale, which, as usual, was begging for attention on the floor against my bedroom wall. My heart dropped as the number, unchanged from the day before, taunted me. Then it was her turn; same thing, no weight loss.

After exchanging a few choice expletives, we looked at each other and silently made a decision. The scale was now the enemy. We snatched it up, marched outside, and negotiated who would get to throw it on the ground and destroy it.

I lived on one of those quintessential pre-war, suburban streets where an ice cream truck comes along every afternoon. You borrow sugar from your neighbor and wave as everyone you know drives by. Sure enough, at that exact moment, one of my neighbors stopped in front of my house in her SUV to say hello. Seeing us holding the scale with determination, she slid her sunglasses down her nose curiously. When we told her our intentions, she gladly became our coconspirator.

We placed the scale just behind the back tire—and with a roar of the engine, what happened next seemed to be in slow motion. She threw the car into reverse and drove over the scale. There was a satisfying crunch as it shattered. We cheered, and everything we thought we knew about finding ourselves by chasing a number was crushed into a thousand shiny pieces.

After 20 years, I was finally free! Free of deciding whether I'd step on the scale with my clothes on or off, my shoes on or off; on the tile, the wood, or the carpet; before a bowel movement or after; on my period or not; after I went out to dinner or in the morning.

I wanted to lose weight so I could love the body I was in. But what I lost on that weight-loss journey was the opportunity to love myself *first*. The day I got off the scale was the beginning of finding that love. I stopped thinking about the number and started thinking about my whole body, mind, and self. I stopped following the diets, and I started listening to what my body wanted and needed to thrive. I stopped dedicating myself to the most challenging exercise programs I could find and started aligning my exercise and lifestyle with how I wanted to feel every day. I dedicated myself to learning as much as I could about the physical body and the subtle energy we all can feel for a lifetime of health instead of a temporary weight loss. As a result, I received something greater. I tapped into an energetic vibration that brought me more love and joy, clarity, closer relationships, security, and emotional well-being.

You're likely reading this because you're curious about finding freedom from dieting. You want to learn what it feels like to eat to fuel your body. You want to be more consistent with your choices. You want to heal past or present inflammatory illnesses or avoid future ones altogether. You want to stop thinking about the next diet, and the next diet, and the next diet.

You also might want to lose weight—and that's okay. But you can have so much more when you let go of that outcome.

Choosing a diet today feels like standing in the cereal aisle, overwhelmed by endless options. Do you go for the all-natural one? The sugar-free one? The one with the fewest calories? The one packed with protein? Or the one loaded with fiber? Maybe you skip them all because you're fasting. It's enough to make you throw your hands up and say, "F— it, I'll just eat whatever I want!" And even though we genuinely want to feel good, we often make choices that leave us feeling guilty instead.

So, what food choices truly serve our best interests and help us reclaim our power? They are the ones that work with our bodies, not against them. The choices that nourish us first on a physical level—energizing, sustaining, and supporting our well-being—and then, as a result, bring emotional satisfaction, not guilt.

This book is for women who want to live boldly beyond dieting. If you're ready to stop stepping on the scale to measure your self-worth and to have tangible results for a lifetime of joy in your body, I will teach you how through *Energetic Eating*. By the end of this book, you will get off the scale and learn how to listen to what your body needs and take action from a place of self-love.

Now, I want you to imagine two different ways of being.

Way 1: You want to lose weight. Every day, you tell yourself how much you hate what you see in the mirror, hoping it will motivate you to make "good" choices. You avoid pictures or make sure you're in the back. You step on the scale to see the progress you've made, the damage you've done, or how far you have to go. You search for a diet to control the situation, hoping it will finally work this time.

How does that feel? Heavy, hard, stuck, frustrating? It's when we become hyper-fixated on the one part of ourselves we want to change. It's what we are taught every day by diets that commodify women's body negativity. It's the energy of loss—and what happens when we take action for only one reason: seeking a specific number on a scale.

That's the energy of weight loss—an energy of negativity and scarcity.

Way 2: Every day, taking action feels effortless because you choose to see yourself as healthy and strong. You're motivated to make changes beyond weight loss, driven by a desire for a life that feels easier, more joyful, and deeply fulfilling. You're front and center in photographs—no more hiding, no more fidgeting with your clothes. You don't need the scale to tell you how you feel; you're already confident in your body, your choices, and the life you're creating.

How does that feel? That's Energetic Eating. It's an energy of positivity, empowerment, and joy.

That's the energy you get to be in today. You get to choose that energy and take action from a place of power and self-love. It's an energy you create—it's not given to you in a diet plan or a number on the scale—it's experienced *within* you.

The key isn't finding the right diet or reaching for the right weight, but aligning the powerful thoughts, foods, and lifestyle to support *you*. Anyone can follow a list of foods for a few weeks. Anyone can step on a scale. That's a diet. I will guide you through how to listen to your body to discover what *you* need, and not just for 30 days. For a lifetime.

I will teach you the Triad of Health—how you "Think," "Eat," and "Live"—to help you understand what your unique body utilizes to thrive. Together, we will generate a vision for the person you want to be in the world, a vision I call your Best Energetic Self. Then, I will support you as you identify and release core memories related to body image and dieting. Once you've identified your history with body image and dieting and understand the negative impacts of fad dieting, we will explore the Six Pillars of Energetic Eating: Thoughts, Mood, Digestion, Focus, Energy Levels, and Conscious Choices.

I'll walk you through how to listen to your body step-by-step. In the future, if you ever feel disconnected or need a reminder, you can visit the portal or any pillar in this book as a reference.

Welcome to *Energetic Eating*—a space where diet confusion dissolves and we rediscover our innate connection to nourishment and well-being. Here, we challenge outdated beliefs and embark on a journey toward lasting freedom that transcends food. *Energetic Eating* isn't simply a way to eat; it's an invitation to live with purpose, alignment, and deep fulfillment. By tuning in to your body's subtle signals and honoring its natural rhythms, you'll find that the wisdom you gain not only transforms your relationship with food but enriches every aspect of your life. Embrace this moment to step into the healthiest, most empowered version of yourself.

PART I:
THE ENERGETIC EATING METHOD

CHAPTER 1

THE FIVE COMMITMENTS

In the twenty years that I chose dieting over listening to my body, I didn't spend a single second *loving* my body. I'd just look in the mirror, step on the scale, and take daily pictures to track changes. I'd tug at my body fat and mentally plan what *not* to eat. I felt the same about being a size 18 as I did about a size 10. Nothing was ever good enough.

Like many other women, I felt unworthy and like a failure if I didn't follow the diet and a false sense of security if I did—successful even, but only if I followed it and lost weight. This kept me stuck in a cycle of yo-yo dieting and decades of losing and gaining the same 30 pounds over and over again.

We have been taught to reduce our wonderfully complex bodies to a number on a scale. You may have devoted vast amounts of time and thought to finding the right diet to lose weight. The fact is that, by doing this, you have been missing out on what it's like to live in harmony with the body you have.

Based on my experience and that of the hundreds of women who I have worked with, I have found that all women who are stuck in the typical cycle of yo-yo dieting tend to take on five false beliefs perpetuated by the multibillion-dollar dieting industry about what they need to lose weight. We will address these five beliefs now and reframe them so that we can clear our subconscious of these harmful messages.

The subconscious mind is like a powerful storage system for all of our beliefs, habits, and past experiences. It operates beneath our conscious awareness, influencing how we think, feel, and behave without us even realizing it. When we repeatedly hear messages, especially from pervasive sources within our culture, our subconscious absorbs and stores them as truths, even if they are harmful or false. Over time, these beliefs become deeply rooted and shape how we perceive ourselves and our ability to achieve our goals—like weight loss. Clearing these memories from your subconscious will help you energetically align yourself to the thoughts, nutrition, and lifestyle that serve you best, which we will address one by one in the coming chapters. For now, let's identify and clear these beliefs.

The Five False Beliefs

- **Measurement:** I need to measure joy in a number rather than look for joy within myself.
- **Negativity:** I need to use negative self-talk to motivate myself to take action.
- **Procrastination:** I need to lose weight before I live my life fully.
- **Comparison:** I need to compare myself to others in order to change.
- **Blame:** I need to rely on a diet rather than myself.

If any of these feel true for you, you're not alone. I used to think I needed weight loss to help me let go of the frustration on the scale and the shame about my body. But it wasn't until I learned to replace these negative beliefs with self-compassion that I discovered my true path to health, healing, and a natural, stable weight.

Today, I encourage my clients to live by the *Five Commitments* rather than be at the mercy of the false beliefs. To take the first step toward freedom, I encourage you to read the following commitments to yourself aloud.

The Five Commitments

Measurement:

I no longer need the scale to determine my value. To release myself from seeking joy on the scale and find freedom in choosing what is best for me, I give myself full permission to experience health without a number.

Negativity:

I recognize when I speak unkindly to myself, and I reframe the thoughts that keep me stuck ruminating, worrying, or judging my body. I take action based on what I truly want for a powerful and healthy life, not based on a sense of lack or a number on the scale.

Procrastination:

I trust my instincts and take action now. I no longer put off starting anything until a later date. Starting today is the most powerful tool. I am brave enough to take imperfect action.

Comparison:

There is a unique plan that works for me and my body. I can tune in to what each of my choices means in the moment and let myself experiment with those choices without comparing myself to my past self or others.

Blame:

I take full responsibility for the choices I make in my life without blaming myself, time, money, or others. I am in charge of my own body and am willing to listen to how my body feels rather than judge it by a number.

To begin to rewire the negative beliefs into positive commitments, I urge you to stop weighing yourself and read or repeat the commitments that resonate with you for up to 21 days. This will be a huge first step in escaping the dieting cycle. As you become more aware of when you are engaging with false beliefs, remember the commitments you've made with yourself to change them. You will start to feel lighter and freer from these limitations and will open yourself up to the journey of *Energetic Eating* through listening to your body.

The Problem with Fad Dieting

Why do women turn to fad diets? The women I work with aren't just consumed with body image and weight loss. They are driven, passionate women who want to feel at home in their bodies so they can focus on what truly matters. But the pressure to *fix* their weight quickly leads them to chase solutions that promise fast results. They ask themselves, *How can I lose weight? What are other women doing? What's the most effective method? What will take the least amount of time?*

This constant search keeps them stuck in the cycle of dieting—always looking for the next solution, only to end up feeling frustrated, defeated, and disconnected from their own needs. The problem isn't a lack of effort; it's that most diets set women up to fail. To break free, we need to first understand why these common diets keep us trapped in self-doubt and disappointment. Let's take a closer look at the patterns behind them and why they don't work.

- **Calorie Counting:** This method of surplus and deficit, which hyper-focuses on food and exercise, ignores important principles of nutrition that help us avoid overeating, indulging in processed foods, and binging due to feeling deprived. It pays little to no attention to nutritional value, and makes it difficult to learn to listen to your body's natural signals. It trains us to believe that if we eat the right amount of calories, we've done a good job; if we don't, we've done a bad job. It values only weight loss and keeps us in a scale-focused mentality. We take action from lack (fewer calories) as opposed to abundance (more nutrition).
- **Carb Counting:** Carbs are not the only relevant consideration when making choices for our health. Non-alcoholic drinks and alcoholic drinks might have the same amount of carbohydrates, but only one of them will give you a hangover. A "carb-conscious" protein bar might have a lower carb count but contains harmful ingredients like sugar alcohols or stabilizing ingredients that disrupt gut health. Contrary to what carb-counting diets claim, fueling your body with whole-food carbohydrates is often more beneficial than consuming processed, low-carb alternatives.
- **Protein Counting:** A protein-centered diet may seem like the answer for women trapped in yo-yo dieting, but it often backfires when approached with the same restrictive mindset. While protein supports satiety and muscle maintenance, prioritizing it at the expense of fiber, healthy fats, and complex carbs can lead to nutrient imbalances, sluggish digestion, and hormonal disruptions. Too much

protein with too few carbs can raise cortisol levels, slowing metabolism and increasing cravings, making long-term adherence difficult.

- **Pre-packaged meals:** Microwavable, pre-packaged meals may seem like an easy solution for weight loss, but these meals are typically highly processed, low in fiber, and designed for calorie control rather than true nourishment. Many contain preservatives, artificial ingredients, sugar alcohols, and excessive sodium, which can lead to bloating, blood sugar crashes, and cravings—making it harder to maintain balanced eating long-term.

As you can see, a lot of the problems with fad diets are that they are black and white, focusing on numbers and restriction rather than mindful eating and sustainable habits. Instead of adhering to rigid diet rules and restrictions like this, which inhibit the ability to make healthy decisions for ourselves, we can cultivate a deeper connection with our bodies to inform us of the choices we can make to feel healthier. I know that with other priorities in your life, it can be tempting to choose something that seems as simple, quick, and straightforward as a fad diet. But the danger is that we fail to make the connection between food and our bodies—we have been led to believe we aren't smart enough to know what's good for our bodies and what's not. But we can tune into our bodies to know when and what to eat, discerning when we need more vegetables, fruits, carbohydrates, healthy fats, and protein. *Energetic Eating* empowers us to tap into our innate wisdom.

Let me share a personal anecdote from about 12 years ago. At that time, I meticulously tracked my food and weight and used a system that gave me a detailed breakdown of macronutrients. I recall feeling anxious about every meal I made for myself: Would I put dressing or yogurt on my sandwich wrap? How many calories were in my wrap? I was constantly measuring portions.

It was a daily struggle to keep up with it, and I was getting sick of all the tracking. I felt like I had more important things to do than micromanage my food. When the scale didn't reflect my desired weight loss, I'd stop meticulously tracking and give up, spiraling into a cycle of self-blame and emotional eating. I felt moody, bloated, and had energy crashes. These were signs I was ignoring my body's signals.

I was sending my body a cascade of harmful messages: that my happiness hinged on weight loss, that the numbers were more important than the way I felt, and that I didn't know how to nourish myself. I was blocking my own potential for health and well-being.

If I could go back in time, here's what I would tell my younger self:

You get to feel healthy today. Your body is not a math equation of surpluses and deficits, nor a machine that requires relentless monitoring and calculation. It is a living, breathing expression of you—worthy of care, joy, and freedom. You deserve more than the exhaustion of chasing a number on the scale. What if, instead of choosing the next diet, you chose to value yourself as you are right now? You'd nourish yourself from a place of trust, make choices that feel good, and finally step off the hamster wheel of self-doubt. Your healthiest life isn't waiting on the other side of restriction—it's available to you the moment you decide you're already enough.

Women who choose diets over listening to their bodies often focus on calorie counting, high-fat or high-protein diets, or tracking their food intake at the cost of *listening* to what their bodies need. Conversely, women who achieve lasting success don't focus on tracking their intake. They have learned how to listen to their bodies' signals. I know because I have taught hundreds of women to do just this—and watched them rediscover freedom, joy, and purpose while also achieving their health goals.

By adopting the principles of *Energetic Eating*, you are about to discover how to interpret your body's unique language, see yourself in a new light, and experience the same empowering transformations as my clients.

They tell me things like:

- "I am the boss of me."
- "I truly feel present in the moment with myself."
- "I realize it's okay to carve out time for myself."
- "The weight came off and I learned to love myself in the process."
- "Exercising and eating well doesn't feel hard anymore. It's just part of who I am."

If you want to love yourself, that work starts now. The most authentic version of yourself emerges when you make choices in alignment with how much you listen to your body and love yourself today, *not* how many pounds you want to lose. It's time to learn to do that.

Let's dive in. In the next chapter, I will uncover the power of integrative nutrition and energy healing and introduce you to the Triad of Health.

CHAPTER 2

THE TRIAD OF HEALTH

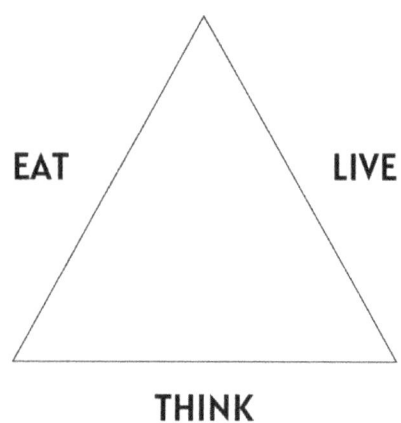

Before I studied integrative nutrition and energy healing, I believed health boiled down to two things: eating what I thought I should and exercising according to the latest diet trend. As a high achiever committed to going all in, I often fell into all-or-nothing thinking. This mindset kept me striving and falling short, trapped in a cycle of pressure and self-judgment. No matter how hard I tried, the perpetual sense of "failure" overshadowed my efforts.

After I ran over my scale in 2018, I knew it was time for a new approach. I enrolled in the Institute for Integrative Nutrition to study how food supports whole-person health. Through this journey, I discovered that true health goes beyond weight loss—it's about nourishment on every level. I began taking steps to reduce inflammation and improve my overall well-being, not just through what was on my plate, but through the holistic idea of "primary food"—the relationships, movement, purpose, and joy that feed us just as much as nutrition does. I also deepened my connection to my "why" for choosing health and learned to honor what truly helped my body thrive—aligning with the life I was living rather than chasing a number.

The following year, I discovered energy kinesiology, a transformative practice that revealed the deeper layers of my health issues. I studied at The Kinesiology Institute, learning how the body's subtle energies influence physical and emotional well-being. Through muscle testing, a technique that assesses the body's response to gentle pressure on specific muscles, I began uncovering blockages in energy reflected in the body's responses. These subtle shifts mapped areas of unresolved stress or misalignment, offering a pathway to the root causes of inflammation and stress in my body.

Each muscle's responsiveness provides insights into one's emotional and physical systems, including beliefs, food sensitivities, and stress on organs and muscles. Through the subdiscipline of biochemical kinesiology, I identified the exact foods that disrupted my digestion, while psychological kinesiology illuminated the limiting beliefs driving my restrictive behaviors and self-judgment. These explorations revealed to me the transformative power of touch with acupressure and tapping, easing discomfort and inviting a sense of relief into the body. This work became central to my healing journey, as I began releasing deep-rooted patterns and embracing a new way of living.

As various deep-seated blocks dissolved, I experienced a profound shift. For the first time, rather than following a list of foods, I could fully listen to my body's needs and honor its signals without falling back into the trap of fad dieting. I'd learned firsthand that true healing requires addressing integrative and energetic aspects of health. It wasn't just about changing what I ate—it was about deeply understanding how to think, eat, and live in alignment with my health.

As I began treating women seeking weight loss through this framework, the deeper roots of their struggles quickly became clear. Their weight gain wasn't just about food—it was very often linked to imbalances in their thoughts, mood, digestion, focus, energy levels, and ability to make conscious choices. The real transformation happened when we addressed these core issues through mindset, nutrition, and lifestyle—what I call the *Triad of Health*. By shifting their approach from restriction to restoration, they began to experience lasting change—not just on the scale, but in how they felt every day.

When the COVID-19 pandemic brought in-person sessions to a standstill, I had to rethink how to guide women without the hands-on feedback of muscle testing. This challenge became an opportunity—I honed a deeper practice of listening to my clients by creating a safe space online where women could fully express themselves. Over time, I learned to recognize the imbalances through conversation alone, tuning into the nuances of their words, symptoms, energy, and emotions. Without ever meeting in person, we worked together to shift their mindset, nutrition, and lifestyle in powerful, lasting ways to resolve the imbalances—proving that true transformation isn't about physical proximity, but about deep connection and understanding. We shifted the focus away from traditional weight-centered goals toward an empowering, whole-body approach. We aligned conscious choices with a vision of their healthiest selves, nurturing their well-being on every level.

In my work, I have found that the Triad of Health—how we Think, Eat, and Live—is the foundation of both integrative and energetic well-being. Strengthening this triad isn't about rigid rules; it's about making choices that align with who you truly are—what I call your Best Energetic Self. Throughout this book, you'll see this theme emerge again and again. In the next chapter, we'll dive into creating a vision for your Best Energetic Self and explore how the Triad of Health can guide you toward fully embodying it

.

CHAPTER 3

YOUR BEST ENERGETIC SELF

Starting today, your objective is no longer a number on a scale—it's the vision of who you want to be. Imagine yourself six months from now, thriving in your physical and emotional well-being. The goal is to connect with your aspirations for yourself and your life. In my work with clients, I've noticed that when they direct their energy toward nurturing the most important parts of themselves, they take consistent, meaningful action. However, when their focus shifts solely to their weight, their efforts tend to be short-lived. This happens because connecting with our passions and deepest desires creates choices that resonate with the whole body, mind, and self. In contrast, fixating on your weight can block energy, reinforcing physical limitations, self-doubt, and dissatisfaction. Inevitably, it leaves us unmotivated and unable to take meaningful action.

In the following exercise, we will zoom out and take stock of what we will call your "Best Energetic Self." This is a key first step in building your vision. In our first journaling exercise, I invite you to write freely, expressing everything you desire in the *present* tense, as if it's already happening, using "I am" instead of "I will."

Focus on all aspects of your life and its overall quality instead of weight-based goals. Think about your personal well-being in relation to your career, your home, your travels, your relationships, your spirituality, and your health. For example, if you want to earn

$100,000 per year, you might write, "My health gives me the confidence to set boundaries, ask for a raise, and not worry about future health bills." If you desire a more organized home, you could write, "Stress is manageable in my life. Keeping things organized feels easy. My home is a place to relax, unwind, and connect with myself, friends, and my family." If weight loss is a goal, emphasize the positive outcomes: "Exercise helps me feel at home in my body. I run around with my kids and happily pose for pictures. I am strong and honor my body daily with nourishing foods. I choose my outfits with joy and feel confident in my clothes."

Your journey back to yourself starts and ends with envisioning what you truly want in your abundant and amazing life. I revisit this exercise myself and with my clients at least four times a year. Now, let's envision what I call your Best Energetic Self.

Your Best Energetic Self

Imagine I could wave a magic wand and instantly grant you your ideal health. Picture yourself six months from now—feeling, vibrant, energetic, confident, and completely at ease in your body. How do you feel? What does your daily routine look like? What choices are you making? Use the three sections provided to explore different facets of your transformation.

Career, work, service, finances:

Relationships, home, travel, intimacy:

Health, spirituality, home-cooking, exercise:

Creating a vision for your life is a powerful process that *elevates your mindset and strengthens your sense of purpose.*, opening you up to new possibilities instead of keeping you stuck in a cycle of fad dieting and disappointment. When you envision your desires in the present tense, you shift from a state of wanting to one of certainty. This clarity allows you to do exactly what you want for yourself and ignites the drive to pursue it every day.

Before I envisioned my Best Energetic Self, I was stuck in a cycle of weighing myself, counting calories, and obsessing over macros. I so desperately desired a specific number on the scale. But when I envision my Best Energetic Self, here is what's different: I am writing about *who* I want to be, not the body I want to have. Imagining your ideal self and the positive outcomes you will create—comfort, strength, love, and fulfillment—deeply connects your motivation to change your soul energy instead of weight-loss energy.

Applying the Triad of Health to your Best Energetic Self

At the heart of the Triad of Health—Think, Eat, and Live—is your Best Energetic Self. When you align these three elements, you tap into a state of harmony. Instead of chasing external fixes, true health emerges from the synergy of cultivating a resilient mindset, nourishing your body, and living in a way that keeps you connected to your deeper purpose. Let's explore this in more detail.

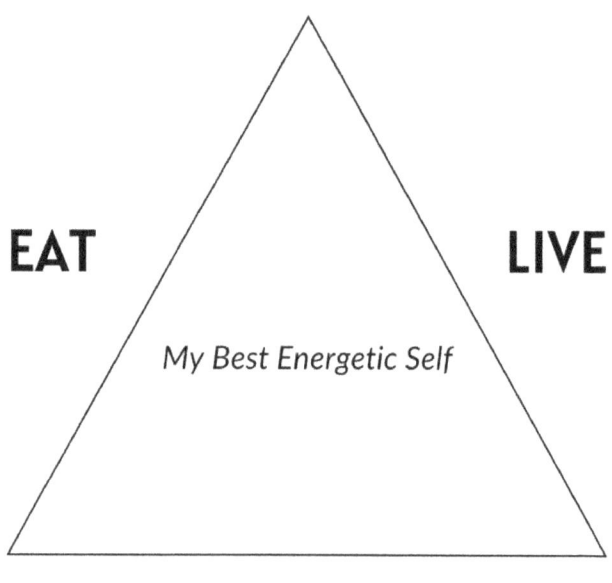

How we Think

Our thoughts form the foundation of the triad. The ways we perceive our bodies and the thoughts we have about ourselves profoundly impact our overall health, either limiting or supporting us. By learning to train our minds, release limiting beliefs, and reframe negative thought patterns, we can learn to make conscious, in-the-moment decisions that support our Best Energetic Selves.

How we Eat

The food we consume carries energy that nourishes or depletes us. It's not simply about good foods or bad foods, but rather about prioritizing nutrition that resonates with the body, supporting how we want to feel. It's about counteracting limitations, like inflammatory stress, that can make us feel sick or unwell. By tuning into our own signals, we can learn to sense the impact of different foods on our Best Energetic Selves.

How we Live

Lifestyle factors such as stress management, adequate sleep, and regular physical activity play a crucial role in supporting hormonal balance, promoting cellular regeneration, boosting metabolism, and optimizing energy flow for our Best Energetic Selves.

When these three parts of the triad work in harmony, our bodies feel stronger, lighter, and more aligned. When one of them is compromised, we can feel weaker and heavier. We might feel like something is broken, blocking the feel-good energy in our bodies. We might feel imbalances in the Six Pillars of Health that we will explore in the following chapters such as negative thought patterns, moodiness, digestive difficulty, lack of focus, lethargy, and trouble making conscious choices towards feeling good. But we have the power to shift that energy. We have the power within us to listen to our bodies and heal the Triad of Health.

Here's how the Triad of Health can play a role in impacting our daily choices and overall well-being:

- We eat something that makes us feel unwell, and then we feel guilty for making that choice. Both the "Eat" and "Think" parts of the triad are broken. When both of those are broken, it's more likely that we will choose not to exercise today (impacting the "Live" part of the triad). All of the parts of the triad are broken.
- We don't wake up early to work out, and the guilt comes in. Now, both the "Live" and the "Think" parts of the triad are broken. It's harder to eat well. The whole triad is broken.
- We wake up with anxious thoughts (Think) and then choose to satisfy them with food (Eat). At this point, we might skip our workout because we feel so guilty that we don't think we can do it (Live). All parts of the triad are broken.

Instead of healing the imbalance within the triad, we let the entire foundation collapse. In these moments, we grasp for diets, unaware that the triad itself is broken—we don't see the deeper issue; we only see our perceived failure. *Energetic Eating* helps you strengthen the Triad of Health and make conscious choices based on how you feel each day, so you know what support your body needs emotionally, nutritionally, and physically. A healthy triad means a healthy life. Imagine if the Triad of Health was working for you instead of against you:

- We eat something that makes us feel unwell. We treat this neutrally as data that lets us know that different choices would make us feel better. We don't feel guilty for eating it; we feel empowered by our own knowledge. This keeps us from breaking the "Think" part of the triad. We decide to move on without guilt and exercise without shame or blame, being gentle with ourselves so we don't break the "Live" part of the triad either. The triad is easier to repair, and we don't feel so broken that we need to look for a diet.
- We don't wake up early to exercise even though we'd planned to. The "Live" part of the triad feels broken. But we give ourselves grace and think about what's possible today even if we didn't wake up early—perhaps a 20-minute midday walk or a quick yoga video online. We eat a good breakfast. Even though the "Live" part of the triad might have felt broken, we've done our best to repair it and kept the other parts strong. It repairs easily, so we don't feel desperate for a diet.
- We wake up with anxious thoughts. Even though we feel this way, we know that exercising, meditating, and eating well will help us feel better. The anxious thoughts dissipate because of self-care. The "Think," "Eat," and "Live" parts of the triad remain intact. We feel close and in tune with our bodies rather than pulled to a diet to fix ourselves.

These examples highlight the deep connection among the elements of the Triad of Health, each working together to support your Best Energetic Self. Now, we'll explore the Six Pillars of Health—Thoughts, Mood, Digestion, Focus, Energy Levels, and Conscious Choices—which serve as messengers, signaling when something is out of energetic alignment and guiding us toward what needs healing. By understanding how these pillars support the Triad of Health, we can break free from the cycle of dieting. The Six Pillars pathway is represented in a graphic, and will highlight the pillar we are addressing in each chapter.

THE SIX PILLARS OF ENERGETIC EATING

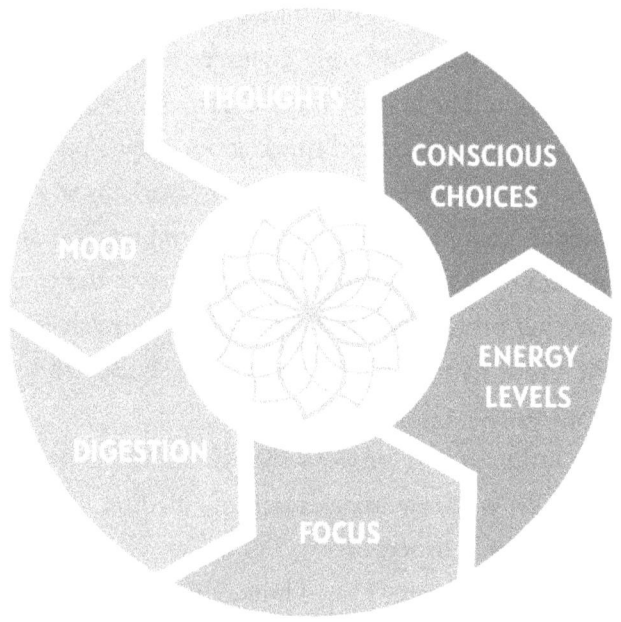

Supporting your Best Self with the Six Pillars of Health

When I started asking myself, "*How do I want to feel today to support my Best Energetic Self?*" and not, "*How much weight do I want to lose?*" I broke free from the endless cycle of dieting and empowered myself to listen to what my body truly needed. The truth is that weight loss alone often isn't important enough to motivate us to make sustainable change. We are complex, dynamic, unique individuals with dreams and wishes that extend far beyond weight-loss goals. As we saw in the Best Energetic Self exercise, we each have a vision within us for a more powerful life.

Next, we will assess how you feel based on the Six Pillars of *Energetic Eating*: Thoughts, Mood, Digestion, Focus, Energy Levels, and Conscious Choices. The *Energetic Eating* pillars are intentionally presented in this order so that you begin with the foundational elements that support your overall well-being and end with the ability to make conscious choices.

Every pillar has its own chapter that will:

- Teach you the role each pillar plays in your health.
- Help you assess your health within the pillar.
- Connect to the "Think," "Eat," and "Live" parts of the triad.
- Give you tools to help you make conscious choices for your Best Energetic Self.
- Include short exercises (called Quick Looks) that reinforce the core concepts and help you instill lasting change.
- Provide examples of the power of conscious choices within the pillar.
- Include downloads and bonus resources.

You can also use this book as a valuable reference, guiding you back to balance within any pillar as needed. Remember, listening to your body and nourishing it with the insights you will learn in the upcoming chapters are the keys to maintaining a strong Triad of Health and supporting your Best Energetic Self.

PART II:
THE SIX PILLARS OF ENERGETIC EATING

CHAPTER 4

PILLAR 1: YOUR THOUGHTS

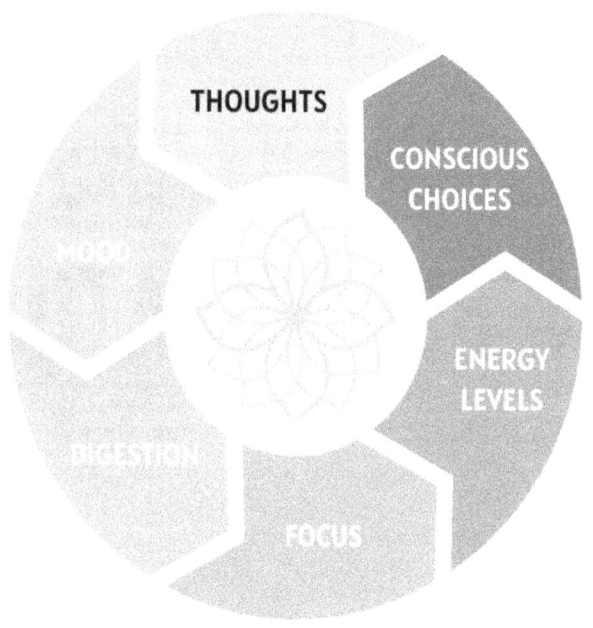

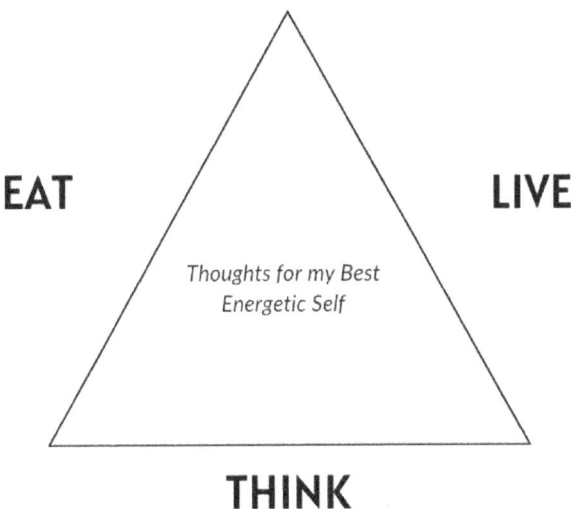

In this chapter, we will examine the Think part of the triad, and explore the affirmation, "There is a unique plan for me." Thoughts and affirmations will guide us to the Eat and Live parts of the triad in later chapters. For now, we will focus only on Think.

Overview

Your thoughts can carry an energy to fuel your health and happiness, guiding you toward the choices that align with how you want to feel. While most diets emphasize willpower, *Energetic Eating* teaches you that shifting your thoughts—releasing negative beliefs and instilling empowering ones—is the one of the keys to unlocking conscious choices that support your Best Energetic Self. Our thoughts about the situations we face shape our feelings, which drive us to take action—or not. These actions then reinforce the beliefs we hold about ourselves, which, in turn, influence our next thoughts. This cycle makes our thoughts incredibly powerful, which is why they're a part of the triad *and* a key pillar. Without addressing our thoughts in a holistic way, we risk blindly following rules and steps that don't align with our personal experiences, leading to resistance and hindering meaningful behavior change.

Thoughts Reflection

Rate each of the following on a scale of 1–5, with 1 meaning "never," 3 meaning "sometimes," and 5 meaning "always."

Consider the following questions over the last six months:

- Do you have recurring negative thoughts about your body?
- Do you believe diets will fix your relationship with your body?
- Do you find yourself feeling out of control around food?
- Do you ever avoid shopping for clothes because of your body?
- Do you feel anxious about attending social events due to fear of judgment?

Total: ___ out of 25

As you fill out the assessment in this chapter and the following chapters, remember there is no judgement here regardless of whether you scored a 5 or a 25! Have grace with yourself—and that is true for all the reflection you'll be doing in this book. No matter what number you scored, you likely have room to improve your thoughts, so I encourage you to explore and implement the suggestions in the rest of the chapter. If you scored 15 or more, the suggestions in this chapter will be important for you to explore and implement. We will delve into the affirmations, nutrition, and lifestyle practices that will support a more positive relationship with yourself and your body.

Affirmations

Choosing and cultivating thoughts that serve us rather than limit our potential is one of the most profound shifts we can make to heal the body and a step you can make today. Even if weight loss is a goal, we can find motivation in what's going well in our lives rather than targeting what we hate about our bodies.

Diets often perpetuate negative self-talk—remember the five false beliefs we discussed earlier? They encourage us to follow the rules instead of trusting our bodies, to focus on setbacks instead of successes, and to compare ourselves to our past selves and others instead of embracing who we are. This is why we must begin with thoughts, bringing awareness to our mindset and how it affects our eating and behavior patterns.

This is where the 12 Positive Affirmations of *Energetic Eating* come into play. They are empowering statements that lead to the actions you need to set yourself free from diets. I crafted them based on years of listening to women's struggles with body image and the deep-seated limiting beliefs that prevented them from listening to their bodies' natural cues. Positive affirmations rooted in confidence help replace limiting beliefs rooted in fear and negativity.

Before we delve into the positive ones, I want you to read the negative affirmations below. If these resonate with you, use the positive affirmations to help you shift your energy, let go of dieting, and fully embrace whole-body health. As you read the negative beliefs, notice how your body responds—perhaps your posture slumps, your face tightens into a frown, or you sense tension or stress building within. This physical reaction reflects the impact of diet beliefs on your energetic body.

The 12 Negative Affirmations

1. I have to choose the right diet plan.
2. I can't commit to my health right now.
3. Losing weight is more important than listening to my body.
4. I only choose foods to help me lose weight.
5. Exercise doesn't count unless I go all in.
6. I always fall off the wagon.
7. I trust the diet more than I trust myself.
8. My body is broken.
9. I have to power through my day.
10. It's not possible for me to choose health when my life is chaotic.
11. It's not possible for me to choose health when I am responsible for the well-being of others.
12. Prioritizing my weight is necessary for me to feel good about myself.

How would you respond if a friend came to you saying these things? Chances are, you'd want to wrap her in a hug and remind her how amazing she is and that she's fully supported. You'd reassure her that she isn't broken and encourage her to be kinder to herself. You might even suggest exploring a more balanced way of living so she doesn't feel so restricted. What if you offered yourself that same grace?

Now, we are going to read the positive affirmations. Notice how your posture grows taller. You feel more at ease, confident, and excited to make changes.

The 12 Positive Affirmations

1. There is a unique plan for me.
2. I am committed to my health.
3. I respect the rhythm of my body.
4. I choose foods that make me thrive.
5. I am powerful and flexible.
6. I trust my process.
7. I am the creator of my healthy habits.
8. My body is healthy and strong.
9. I know the right action at any given moment.
10. I create an environment in which I can flourish.
11. I cherish my relationships.
12. Prioritizing my health leads to joy and balance.

My clients use these affirmations when they feel stuck, unsure, or drawn into the dieting mindset. We will explore how we can move from negative to positive affirmations in deeper detail throughout this book. For now, I encourage you to familiarize yourself with them, rewrite them, and display them somewhere visible. Writing down and reading these affirmations daily will enhance positive brain activity, reprogram your subconscious mind, and improve your ability to internalize and recall them. By taking a few moments to sit quietly and reflect on these positive affirmations in a relaxed state, you can also tap into the profound power of meditation to deepen their impact. This practice not only calms your mind but also creates the ideal mental environment to heal the subconscious beliefs that keep you trapped in the dieting cycle, paving the way for lasting transformation. Visit the book portal for a guided meditation using these positive affirmations.

Your thoughts will guide you to make conscious decisions about your health and well-being. When you encounter challenges, you may not always be able to get to the grocery store, work out for 40 minutes, or sleep for eight hours. However, you can immediately change your thoughts. That's why, in addition to the pillars, affirmations are threaded throughout the program and linked to the "Think" part of the triad. Remember from Chapter 3 that, if we can repair one part of the triad, we can keep it strong and continue to support our Best Energetic Selves.

Now we will dive into the first affirmation: "There is a unique plan for me." The rest of the affirmations are threaded throughout the remaining pillars of this book.

THINK: *There is a unique plan for me.*

This affirmation is about accepting that there is no single right or wrong way to adopt a health journey. There is a way that is unique to you. Diets want us to believe there is a one-size-fits-all approach, but you are a multi-layered and dynamic individual. As demonstrated through the Best Energetic Self exercise from Chapter 3, you have unique interests and motivations. Your history with dieting and body image informs how you operate and make decisions. These experiences have shaped where you struggle and where you thrive. Therefore, your journey will be unique to you.

Write in a journal or use the space provided to explore what this affirmation means to you.

There is a unique plan for me.

Quick Look: Positive Affirmations

- Write down the positive affirmations and post them in a conspicuous place.
- Reflect on the affirmation, "There is a unique plan for me."
- Visit the book portal for a guided meditation on the 12 Positive Affirmations.

When women come to me distressed about their bodies, I know it always goes deeper than weight loss. They've been so profoundly impacted by fad dieting that they can't envision a way forward without shedding pounds first. It breaks my heart because I know they've lost a part of themselves, a part that was likely stolen from them bit by bit since childhood.

I had a new client who told me she needed "fat camp." I listened intently to all the things she had tried, how hard she had been on herself and all the micromanaging she wanted to do to lose weight despite having me in her corner. In her mind, strict accountability would be the key to finally achieving her weight-loss goal. I waited patiently for her to finish recounting everything that had failed her, then asked, "Why do you think those other approaches have failed?"

She replied, "Because I give it my all, and then I just burn out and don't want to do it anymore."

This is a common cycle. The all-or-nothing mindset keeps so many of us stuck. But where does that mindset come from? What experiences led up to my new client's body dissatisfaction? What was her history with food?

This particular woman grew up in poverty with limited access to food. She described receiving a single quarter a day every summer to buy lunch from the vending machines. For her, food did not provide nourishment. It signaled scarcity. She did not know how to have a consistently positive relationship with food. She viewed herself as someone who couldn't stick to anything and who was constantly sabotaging her own health and weight-loss goals.

But the truth was, she had lifted herself out of poverty. She'd worked tirelessly to get through school, secure a job, start a family, and build a lucrative career. She was safe and didn't need quarters to buy food anymore.

I asked her, "How would it feel to know that food is a safe choice? That you no longer need to worry about where your next meal is coming from or whether you'll have enough to eat?"

Her eyes welled up. "I guess I'd focus more on how I treat myself with food instead of worrying about my body."

"If you stopped worrying about your body, what would change?"

She sat up a little straighter. "I guess I'd just be happy with where I am."

"And if you were happy with where you are, would you do anything differently?"

"I'd still want to take care of myself, but I probably wouldn't be so extreme and hard on myself all the time."

We ended that session addressing her core memories, not with a meal plan, a diet plan, or a list of foods to cut out, but with a plan for how she could love herself more. She began to understand that her choices weren't about being "on" or "off" a diet; they weren't all-or-nothing. They were about the beliefs she'd internalized in childhood that led her to rigidly control her food intake.

I helped her commit to healing her body, not the scale. Together, we built a healthy relationship with her thoughts, food, and lifestyle that she was never taught as a child. No matter your circumstances or experiences, my teaching principles can help you, too. Let's delve deeper into releasing core memories.

Releasing Your Core Memories

In the following exercises, we will explore core memories of dieting, weight gain, and weight loss, identify how these experiences made us feel, and then rethink our beliefs about ourselves. Telling your stories will allow you to reconnect with forgotten parts of yourself that need healing. By identifying and reframing your feelings, you can empower yourself to get unstuck. Not all of the examples in the exercise may resonate with you, and that's okay. Look for themes that feel meaningful to you, and if a specific memory strikes a chord, take the time to answer the questions that follow.

In energy kinesiology, this technique is helpful in releasing all forms of emotional stress, including:

- Fear and anxiety
- Overwhelm
- Disappointment

- Self-Doubt
- Anger and resentment
- Grief and guilt
- Stress from physical pain
- Anxiety
- Regret

You might feel vulnerable sharing these stories for the first time. You might feel sad, angry, or frustrated that these things happened. We must explore the history behind why we do what we do and reframe that history with new thoughts and emotions to let go. Going through this process is never easy, but doing so will help us stop suppressing the pain and feel closer to our Best Energetic Selves. If reflecting on these memories feels too tender or traumatic, or you'd prefer to discuss them with a mental health professional, feel free to skip over them. Do what is best for you.

I will first share an example from my own story, and then I'll invite you to do the same. Through my experience, I will show you how to complete the whole process, and in the exercises that follow, I will prompt you to write about the feelings you had during a specific event and then rewrite your beliefs from an empowered place.

My Earliest Memory of Wanting to Lose Weight

In fifth grade, we had a class project where we were asked to write down our New Year's resolutions. Even at age 10, my first thought was about weight loss. Advertisements had bombarded me with weight loss solutions, and the adults around me reinforced the same message—I had the perfect resolution handed to me before I even knew to question it. But when it came time to share, I remember standing up in the front of the room with all eyes on me—including those of my adoring teacher. It was hard to get the words out. My excitement started to turn to shame.

"I want to lose ten pounds."

It was the first time those words came out of my mouth. And for the first time, I felt embarrassed about my body. Thinking back now, it was the beginning of two decades of repeatedly setting the same intentions, where I stepped on the scale repeatedly to measure my value year after year.

Here is my example of thoughts and beliefs perpetuated by this core memory.

Notice what thoughts and feelings you had in this situation. Write them down below.

Shame, disappointment, self-doubt.

What beliefs were created as a result of these thoughts?

My body is something to be ashamed of. I have to lose weight. I am afraid to love myself.

Review it again. What could you tell yourself about this today?

Your body is perfect. You are strong and resilient. You get to love yourself today.

What positive feelings would you have if that were the case?

Confidence, strength, love.

What beliefs would you have then?

My body is amazing. I am strong. I am capable of loving myself today.

Now it's your turn.

Explore your core memory using the following prompts.

What is your earliest memory of wanting to lose weight? Write down your story.

_____

_____

_____

_____

Notice what thoughts and feelings you had in this situation. Write them down below.

_____

_____

_____

_____

What beliefs were created as a result of these thoughts?

_____

_____

_____

_____

Review it again. What could you tell yourself about this today?

_____

_____

_____

_____

What positive feelings would you have if that were the case?

_____

_____

_____

_____

What beliefs would you have then?

_____

_____

_____

_____

In the rest of the core memories examples, I will only share my stories to inspire you. You will then share your story and answer the prompts in the book or in a journal to release your core memories on your own, without my examples.

Losing Weight

My first big break-up happened when I was fifteen, at the end of my sophomore year of high school. I lost a lot of weight that summer due to the emotional stress. I vividly remember the moment I put on my jean shorts. I recall lying in bed, letting my knees touch, and seeing a gap between my thighs. When I returned to school that fall, I received a compliment I'd never heard before: "Wow, you're so skinny!" I had a newfound confidence and saw myself as popular, likable, and accepted. This became the feeling I looked for over the next two decades.

Release the core memory using the following prompts.

Did you ever lose a lot of weight? What is your earliest memory? Write down your story.

_____

_____

_____

_____

Notice what thoughts and feelings you had in this situation. Write them down below.

_____

_____

_____

_____

What beliefs were created as a result of these thoughts?

_____

_____

_____

_____

Review it again. What could you tell yourself about this today?

_____

_____

_____

What positive feelings would you have if that were the case?

_____

_____

_____

_____

What beliefs would you have then?

_____

_____

_____

My Most Extreme Diet

I embarked on a 7-day fast where I consumed nothing but water, lemon, cayenne, and maple syrup during the day and an absurd amount of salt water first thing every morning to "purge toxins." I remember squeezing the lemons every morning, the acidic citrus juice stinging my fingers. I added the maple syrup as if my life depended on this single source of sustenance to get me through the day.

While drinking the lemonade wasn't so bad taste-wise, the citric acid wreaked havoc on my tooth enamel, causing extreme tooth sensitivity. The salt flush was the worst part; every morning, forcing down this salty concoction that made me gag, followed by running to the bathroom to relieve myself, complete with cramps and uncontrollable diarrhea that ran clear after day four. I went through a fleeting period of elation, but this quickly gave way to flu-like symptoms, headaches, and extreme fatigue, ultimately leading me to abandon the program on day five. Although I lost weight, I gained it all back within two weeks.

Release the core memory using the following prompts.

What was your most extreme diet? Write down your story.

_____

_____

_____

_____

Notice what thoughts and feelings you had in this situation. Write them down below.

_____

_____

_____

_____

What beliefs were created as a result of these thoughts?

_____

_____

_____

_____

Review it again. What could you tell yourself about this today?

___

___

___

What positive feelings would you have if that were the case?

___

___

___

What beliefs would you have then?

___

___

___

Gaining Weight

I stood in line at the weight loss meeting, my heart pounding like I was waiting for the scariest ride at the amusement park. I felt sweaty as I anticipated the dreaded weigh-in, knowing the number on the scale would dictate my allotted points for the week. When my turn finally came, I prepared myself, just like you do for a ride that flips you upside down—taking off my shoes, sweater, and jewelry. But unlike a thrill ride where you want to hold onto your belongings, I prayed I'd lost some weight.

I handed my weight-tracking booklet to the woman in charge of the scale. She held my fate—the number that would tell me what I should believe about myself that day. I stepped on the scale, one foot then the other, closing my eyes. She told me the number: 7 pounds *more* than my last weigh-in. I burst into tears. The number echoed in my head, and I wondered once again how I'd gotten to this point.

Back then, I had zero body awareness and a reckless screw-it mentality. I was disconnected from how my body felt. I was the girl who stood behind her thinner friends in photos and used food and alcohol to soothe herself. After all, my friends seemed able to eat whatever they wanted, so I wasn't sure why I couldn't do the same. But the reality was that most of my friends never had to resort to diets, juice fasts, or calorie restriction. I was the one trapped in a cycle of yo-yo dieting, swinging between indulgence and restriction, and my body was about to endure another round to try and get the weight off.

Release the core memory using the following prompts.

What is one story that stands out about gaining weight? Write down your story.

_____

_____

_____

_____

Notice what thoughts and feelings you had in this situation. Write them down below.

_____

_____

_____

_____

What beliefs were created as a result of these thoughts?

_____

_____

_____

_____

Review it again. What could you tell yourself about this today?

_____

_____

_____

_____

What positive feelings would you have if that were the case?

_____

_____

_____

_____

What beliefs would you have then?

_____

_____

_____

_____

Comments About My Body or Eating

Growing up surrounded by the 90s diet culture and images of gaunt models like Kate Moss in magazines, I was set up to always seek approval from my family and friends about my body and food. I never felt athletic or thin enough compared to my friends and family members. I remember cans of weight loss shakes in my school lunches and being told not to order a chef's salad because it was fattening. It seemed to me that people told me I looked good only when I was thin, and when I wasn't, they made subtle comments about what I should and shouldn't eat or how I should exercise.

Release the core memory using the following prompts.

What do you remember about comments around your body or eating? Write down your story.

_____

_____

_____

_____

Notice what thoughts and feelings you had in this situation. Write them down below.

_____

_____

_____

_____

What beliefs were created as a result of these thoughts?

_____

_____

_____

_____

Review it again. What could you tell yourself about this today?

_____

_____

_____

What positive feelings would you have if that were the case?

_____

_____

_____

What beliefs would you have then?

_____

_____

_____

Now that you have released your core memories with body image and dieting, I want you to see that the way you feel today is not your fault. We are conditioned to see and feel a certain way about our bodies by these core memories, and they create deep-seated beliefs. It is up to us to release these core memories and create a new belief system.

Go back to the exercises where you answered, "What beliefs would you have then?" and then write your new beliefs below.

Writing new beliefs helps reprogram your subconscious mind by replacing limiting or negative beliefs with empowering ones. The act of writing creates a tangible shift and reinforces the new narrative. Then, place your fingertips gently on your forehead until you feel a delicate pulse beneath them. Bring the old memory to mind, and then speak your new beliefs out loud with intention. This helps release the old and integrate the new on a deeper level. To enhance this experience, you can visit the portal for this emotional stress release exercise.

My New Beliefs

Quick Look: Core Memories

- Complete the writing exercise on releasing your core memories.
- Visit the book portal for a guided emotional stress release exercise to release limiting beliefs from your core memories.

The Power of Conscious Choices with your Thoughts

I used to be weighed down by the thoughts I had about myself. It wasn't until I addressed my early experiences with dieting and body image that I was able to let go of the old stories I told myself and adopt new ones.

Today, I consistently envision what is truly important in my life using the Best Energetic Self exercise we did in Chapter 3, and I take action to support that vision instead of dieting. This is possible because I have challenged the negative beliefs I held about myself for so many years. Once I stopped those thoughts from taking over my life, I could listen to what my body needed. You will learn how to do this as we work through the rest of the program's pillars.

As you move through each pillar—whether it's empowering your thoughts, enhancing your mood, supporting digestion, finding focus, balancing energy, or deepening conscious choices—you'll develop an awareness of your body's signals and how to respond with intention. Each pillar will guide you toward making conscious choices that align with your health goals and help you embody your

Best Energetic Self. That's why the pillar "Conscious Choices" comes last—it's where everything comes together, ensuring every choice you make reflects your commitment to your well-being and your highest self.

Energetic Eating Journal

At the end of each pillar, you'll have the opportunity to complete an *Energetic Eating* journaling exercise. This exercise is a key part of my collaborative process with clients—they fill out their journals four times a week in the first few weeks we work together. When clients submit their entries, I review each one with a compassionate eye, guiding them to uncover and challenge their limiting beliefs, nutritional imbalances, and lifestyle factors affecting their Best Energetic Selves. By exploring the underlying "why" behind their choices, we work together to illuminate a clear, empowering path forward.

The journaling process in the context of this book is designed to help you integrate what you've learned and reflect on your conscious choices from every chapter.

We begin by identifying the most important thing ("M.I.T.") you want to focus on to embody your Best Energetic Self. Choose something that feels deeply meaningful to you, something on which you can center your attention for the day. This practice will connect you to the part of yourself that loves who you are becoming rather than fixating on a number on the scale. By honoring your true self in this way, you will create the foundation for lasting, sustainable change. Next, you will reflect on how you can "Think," "Eat," and "Live" in alignment with what you've learned so far, guided by your internal wisdom and the principles from the pillars. Then, you will write down the foods you eat and how they make you feel. This practice encourages mindfulness, helping you slow down and connect your physical sensations to the foods you choose, allowing you to notice what might need adjustment. Finally, you use "Reflections" to celebrate how the conscious choices you made that day positively impacted your Best Energetic Self.

As I guide you through the remaining pillars of Energetic Eating, you will become familiar with additional affirmations (Think), nutrition (Eat), and lifestyle (Live) components that you can incorporate into your journaling. Many of my clients journal daily; others use it for weekly intention setting; and many come back to the practice as needed to remind themselves how to listen and tune into their bodies through *Energetic Eating*.

As I provide the journaling structure and directions, you can download and use the pages from the book portal or rewrite them in your own journal. Choose a time of day that works for you, but most of my clients fill out the "M.I.T." and "Think," "Eat," "Live" sections as an intention in the morning, the foods and feelings section throughout the day, and the "Reflection" section in the evening. Use the prompts to guide you. Blank journal pages and examples of journal entries are available in the portal.

Date: _____

Most Important Thing(s): *What is the most important thing you'd like to focus on from your Best Energetic Self?*		
How I Think:	How I Eat:	How I Live:
What is a positive thought that you would like to take with you?	*When you think about supporting yourself nutritionally, what could that look like now?*	*When you think about supporting yourself through lifestyle choices, what could that look like now?*

Breakfast:	
How did you feel?	

Lunch:
How did you feel?

Dinner:
How did you feel?

Snack 1:	Snack 2:
How did you feel?	How did you feel?

Liquids:
How did you feel?

Reflection: *How are you feeling today? How have these shifts positively influenced your Best Energetic Self?*

CHAPTER 5

PILLAR 2: YOUR MOOD

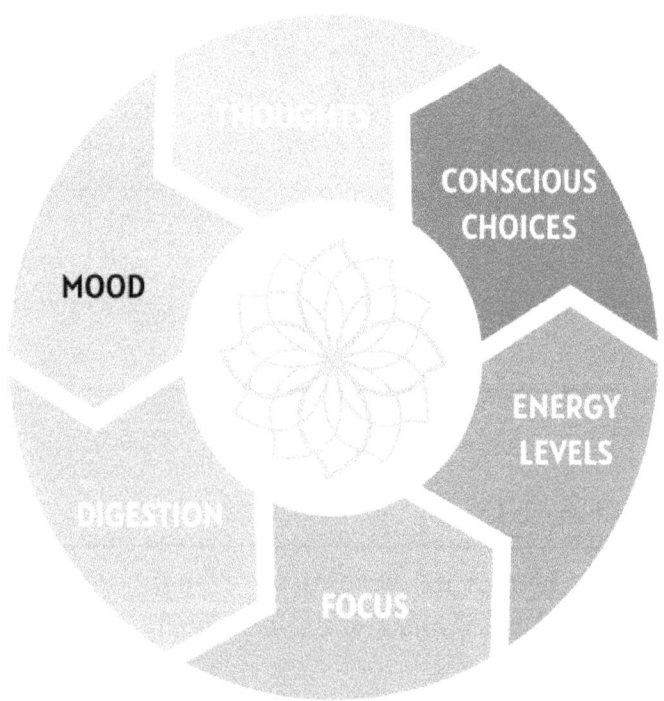

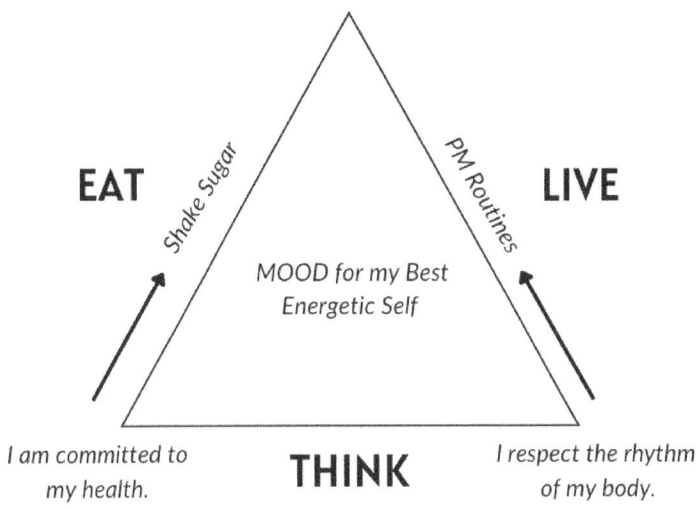

In this chapter, through the Think, Eat, Live Triad, we'll explore two empowering affirmations, a key nutritional component, and a transformative lifestyle shift to support making conscious choices for your mood aligned with your Best Energetic Self.

Overview

Your mood is influenced by a complex interplay of factors, including external circumstances, internal biology, and personal habits. While external events, like stressful situations or unexpected challenges, and internal issues, such as brain chemistry and hormonal changes, can cause us to feel moody, short-tempered, anxious, or depressed, we still hold a significant degree of influence over our mood. By managing blood sugar, cortisol, and stress responses through awareness of hidden sugars and a good evening sleep routine, we can build resilience against mood disruptions. In this chapter, we'll evaluate the impact of moodiness on our Best Energetic Selves and explore affirmations (Think), sugar consumption (Eat), and sleep routines (Live) that will help support our mood.

Mood Reflection

Rate each of the following on a scale of 1–5, with 1 meaning "never," 3 meaning "sometimes," and 5 meaning "always."

Consider these questions in relation to the past six months:

- Do you feel like you're running on empty?
- Do you feel like you're barely holding it together at work and home?
- Is it hard to manage the day without feeling like you want to nap?
- Do you describe yourself as stressed a lot of the time?
- Do you use TV or your devices to wind down at the end of the day?

Total: ___ out of 25

If you scored 15 or higher, the suggestions in this chapter will be especially helpful for you to explore and implement.

Let's look at your first affirmation in this chapter, *I am committed to my health.*

THINK: *I am committed to my health.*

This affirmation is about investing in the bigger picture of your well-being. It's tempting to believe that committing to a diet is the key to health and weight loss, but being committed to your health means focusing on overall health, not just weight. We can accept general guidelines for healthy living without an attachment to the outcome of weight loss. We want to be healthy enough to live longer and make powerful choices for our Best Energetic Selves, which is difficult when we can't manage our moods. Fad diets want us to believe that rigid rules lead to weight loss, but I want you to focus on how openness, curiosity, and learning can lead you to sustainable health.

One of the hardest challenges and a blocker to resolving mood issues is our reliance on sugar, alcohol, and processed food. Evaluating your relationship with these substances is one of the commitments to health that will yield the greatest results for your Best Energetic Self. In this chapter, we'll focus on sugar and alcohol, as I've found they have the biggest effect on our mood and all of the pillars that follow. Remember that the pillars are in a particular order based on impact so you can notice how what you feel affects your Best Energetic Self as quickly as possible.

To overcome mental limitations and your history of committing to diets instead of yourself, use the space provided to journal about what this affirmation means to you.

I am committed to my health.

Now that you've explored what it means to be committed to your health, let's explore the "Eat" portion of the triad as it relates to mood.

EAT: *Shake Sugar and Alcohol*

My Story

When I was 26, I had a drinking habit. Every night, I would either have beer or wine with dinner, followed by an after-dinner drink or a bowl of ice cream. I believed alcohol and a sweet treat was how I could relax, have fun, relate to my partner, and enjoy life.

I tracked my food using points for both food and drinks. The fewer points I consumed, the more weight I was supposed to lose. However, I wasn't consistent with the tracking because I simply didn't want to track my alcohol or evening indulgence. I also couldn't balance my blood sugar due to the alcohol and the foods I ate when my inhibitions were lowered.

This led to off-again, on-again dieting with weight fluctuations up to 20–30 pounds. I lacked consistency with my health because of my evening rituals. I felt bloated and heavy, had low energy, experienced difficulty controlling my emotions, and felt disproportionate anxiety about work tasks.

Maybe you don't consider your drinking or sugar consumption a problem, but even in small amounts, both of these can become subtle dependencies that impact your mood. I've seen it play out not only in my own life but in many of my clients' as well. This up-and-down cycle of blood sugar imbalance affects the brain's immune cells, causing neuroinflammation. As a result, it can cause us to feel irritable, anxious, and worried.

Any feelings of being out of control with sugar or alcohol, like the need to grab a bakery breakfast first thing every morning, aren't actually about the specific foods or drinks. If it were as simple as just avoiding sugar, most of us wouldn't be stuck in the cycle of chasing diets. The key is to address our *relationship* with sugar. Once we start to see our connection with food as a relationship—how we engage with it energetically—we can begin to shift our perspective and make food and lifestyle choices that truly support our Best Energetic Selves.

My unhealthy relationship with sugar and alcohol lasted for years. It wasn't until I stopped trying to control my consumption and started focusing on who I wanted to be as my Best Energetic Self that things shifted. I didn't want to feel physically unwell and moody all the time. I didn't want to feel anxious, depressed, and perpetually out of control around food or dependent on alcohol. I wanted to live powerfully. I knew something had to change, and maybe you do too.

This is why it's important to reflect and take inventory instead of simply declaring that you'll "give it up in the name of weight loss." If you want to stop yo-yo dieting, committing to your Best Energetic Self is the way to get there.

Sugar and Alcohol Inventory

Let's take inventory of your relationship with sugar and alcohol. Write in a journal or use the space provided to reflect on the following questions:

When do you turn to sugar or alcohol for comfort?

_____

_____

_____

_____

How does it impact your mood before, during, and after consumption?

_____

_____

_____

_____

What would you like to change about your relationship with sugar or alcohol?

_____

_____

_____

_____

What would be the first step in doing that?

_____

_____

_____

How would that positively impact your Best Energetic Self?

_____

_____

_____

Understanding your relationship with sugar and alcohol is the first step toward making the changes that I will help you with later in this chapter. You are connecting with the parts of yourself that often go unrecognized, so you can have more self-awareness when it comes to making conscious choices with sugar and alcohol. Now, I will help you understand the impact of sugar and alcohol on the body so you can be deeply invested in your health and well-being for your Best Energetic Self.

Sugar Deep Dive

It's no secret that sugar intake impacts your health, including your weight and your risks of heart disease and diabetes. Many of us have heard this before. The problem is that these facts alone are not enough to get most of us to limit how much we consume or to stop relying on it for a quick fix or mood boost.

It's not entirely our fault; sugar and alcohol are highly addictive, and sugar is hidden in places we don't expect. It is added to food for flavor, to enhance shelf-life, and to stimulate our taste buds. A diet high in refined sugar or alcohol disrupts hormones and causes depression, anxiety, restlessness, nervousness, and impulsivity. You've likely experienced the effects of these highs and lows—it's the craving when avoiding work, or the desire to relax before or after dinner. It's the need for something sweet after lunch when our brains want more stimulation to keep working. It's the impulse for ice cream or a drink when someone lets us down. It's the hankering for a glass of wine when someone else orders one or when we're sitting in front of the TV at the end of a long, stressful, anxiety-ridden day.

To pull it all together, understanding our current relationship with sugar and alcohol is the first step to knowing our starting point. Then, remembering who we want to be as our Best Energetic Selves provides a meaningful reason for cutting back. Finally, understanding how sugar affects the body—its addictive nature and how its negative impact on mood creates a vicious cycle—helps remove shame and self-blame. This is why understanding the science is so important: it shifts the focus from "willpower" to awareness and empowerment. Ironically, feelings like fatigue, cravings, anxiety, and the desire for stimulation aren't relieved by sugar or alcohol; instead, the body needs to be free from them for about a week to start noticing real change. This requires intentionally avoiding refined sugar and alcohol during that time.

You might be thinking, "If it were that simple, I'd have done it already!" I get it—it can feel overwhelming. But I gently challenge that perspective. Now that you've taken inventory of your relationship with sugar, envisioned your Best Energetic Self, and gained a deeper understanding of how sugar and alcohol impacts your body, you're in a much stronger position to cut it out for just one week. For many of my clients, focusing on a single week feels far more manageable than the idea of giving it up forever. Think of it as an experiment: you're collecting valuable data about your body and what it truly needs to thrive. And to truly understand your physiological relationship with sugar, the first step is giving your body a chance to reset by going without it.

How do you reduce sugar cravings? Increase your intake of protein, water, and healthy fats, and swap refined sugar for honey, maple syrup, molasses, or coconut sugar. Women in the *Energetic Eating Method* often ask why I suggest these replacements instead of sugar-free alternatives. The reason is that not all sweeteners are created equal. Low or no-calorie sweeteners can wreak havoc on the gut, and research shows they still trigger an insulin response that disrupts blood sugar levels. By replacing refined sugar with natural sweeteners that have nutritional value, you're building a bridge made of better sugar alternatives from where you are with sugar to where you want to be without a sugar habit.

Most women find that once they make this swap, they crave sweet foods less over time and feel less addicted overall. Incorporating protein with low-glycemic fruits into your diet is a powerful way to curb sugar cravings. Protein keeps you feeling full and satisfied longer, stabilizing your blood sugar and reducing the urge to reach for something sweet. When you pair protein with low-glycemic fruits like berries, apples, or grapefruit, you're nourishing your body with natural sweetness that doesn't spike your blood sugar. In *Energetic Eating*, I often remind women that it's not about deprivation but about committing to your health by giving your body what it truly needs—nutrients that fuel and stabilize you. When you make this shift, you'll notice that cravings for sugar begin to fade, and your body feels more balanced and nourished.

For alcohol cravings, I suggest two things. For an alcohol substitute, add one tablespoon of apple cider vinegar to a glass of water or flavored seltzer. The drink improves gut health and helps the body create a state of equilibrium. A splash of lemon along with the apple cider vinegar will enhance sweetness. You could also replace alcoholic drinks with mocktails or non-alcoholic beer. Just like the sugar swap, even though these drinks have calories, they won't impact your ability to show up as your Best Energetic Self by giving you a hangover. Even one alcoholic drink can disrupt the body in ways we dismiss as "no big deal" despite feeling tired and moody. In my experience, these replacements light up a different part of the brain—one that's willing to have less rather than the part that leaves us wanting more. In a short time, as long as you are committed to your health and reflective about how you want to feel and who you want to be, you'll be empowered to live differently with less sugar and alcohol.

After one week, if you notice your mood has improved and you feel less dependent on sugar, you can reintroduce it in small amounts. Pay close attention to how you feel afterward. If it triggers an addictive response, revisit the affirmation and your free writing exercise: "I am committed to my health."

If you feel moody, short-tempered, or anxious again, view it as valuable insight—it's your body signaling that you've had too much. From there, you have the power to choose: reduce your intake or leave it out altogether. This conscious decision aligns with your Best Energetic Self.

You can repair your relationship with sugar and alcohol. It doesn't always mean cutting them out completely or swearing them off forever—it's about healing the relationship first. Once healed, you can welcome them back in a way that feels good and balanced. You'll know this relationship is healed when you no longer reach for a sweet treat or drink to improve your mood. Instead, you'll feel empowered, making choices that truly serve you rather than being controlled by cravings.

Creating healthy boundaries with sugar and alcohol may initially lead to discomfort. It can be hard when you can't turn to a drink, candy, or a pastry when you are experiencing a negative emotion. However, by not following this urge, you can finally address the underlying issue. Give yourself grace. Remember that sugar and alcohol are addictive, and this change can take time.

Also, remember that even "failures" are successes if you use them as an opportunity to learn and grow. Your body and mind will become more resilient in managing stress and anxiety. For example, if you aren't having your ice cream after dinner in front of the TV, you might realize that you're craving connection with your partner or loved ones. This could motivate you to turn off the TV and reach out. If you eliminate sugar and suddenly find relief from moodiness, digestive issues, gas, and bloating, you might realize you have more power over your well-being than you thought. This newfound empowerment can be scary for some people because when you feel good, discomfort evaporates as an excuse for not taking responsibility for your choices and overall happiness.

For ideas about what to swap with sugar and alcohol, high protein breakfasts to help you start your day with balanced blood sugar, snacks to ward off cravings, and an acupressure tapping exercise to balance blood sugar, refer to the resources below or visit the book portal.

FIND AND REPLACE SUGAR

Pro-tip: Healthy fats such as avocado, nuts, and fish help curb sugar cravings.

Find		Replace
Corn syrup, high fructose corn syrup, tapioca syrup, brown rice syrup, cane juice, evaporated cane juice, fruit juice, fructose, agave	→	Honey, maple syrup
Flavored yogurt	→	Whole-fat greek or plain yogurt topped with fruit & cinnamon
Juice, soda, diet drinks	→	Water, seltzer, flavored seltzer, kombucha, tea
Pastry or muffin	→	Muffins that swap sugar for honey
Granola bar	→	Homemade trail mix with raw nuts, seeds, coconut chips
Cookies	→	Apple with organic natural nut butter
Processed salad dressings	→	Homemade dressing made with olive or avocado oil
Frozen waffles or pancakes	→	Almond-flour and egg-based pancakes

Wine, beer, liquor	→	½–1 tbsp apple cider vinegar in flavored seltzer, honey, squeeze of lemon
Commercially packaged pre-sliced bread	→	Buy fresh sourdough from a bakery, try your sandwich as a salad, or in a collard green wrap
Instant oatmeal	→	Rolled or steel cut oats
Sugar in your coffee	→	Black, with a splash of cream or dairy alternative, and/or with raw honey, date syrup, or maple syrup

LIMITING ALCOHOL		
Habit	→	Do Instead
Most evenings	→	Limit to 2 drinks per week. Then, only on special occasions.
Sugary cocktails	→	Wine or clear hard-alcohol with seltzer and lemon/lime
Your evening ritual	→	Seltzer with ½ tbsp–1 tbsp of apple cider vinegar and a squeeze of lemon. Adding 1 tsp of honey, or ½ a pack of stevia or a stevia drop in the seltzer brings an added satisfying sweetness.
After dinner	→	Choose a hot herbal tea instead.
Ordering a bottle of wine for the table	→	Start with water or seltzer. Order by the glass, alternating with water or seltzer.
Always ordering at a restaurant	→	Try something new and non-alcoholic. Order herbal tea, kombucha (this may have caffeine and impact your sleep) or a fun mocktail.

PROTEIN-BASED BREAKFASTS

Protein-based breakfasts balance your blood sugar and help you feel fuller longer. Your body breaks down proteins into important amino acids that provide energy and enhance satiety.

V. = Vegan

- Full-fat Greek Yogurt Parfait with Purely Elizabeth Granola
  - Nut-milk based yogurt (V.)
- Vegetable Omelet
  - Black beans and rice with avocado and cashew sour cream in a coconut wrap (V.)
- Scrambled eggs and vegetables
- Smoothie or smoothie bowl made with peanut butter, spinach, raspberries, full-fat yogurt and protein powder
  - Nut-milk based yogurt (V.)
- Breakfast pizza with eggs, tomatoes, and cheese on a cauliflower round
  - Scrambled organic tofu or beans, and cheese with vegan cheese or avocado (V.)
- Chia pudding (see recipe in book portal) (V.)
- Cottage Cheese bowl, either with berries for sweet, or tomatoes and black beans for savory (V.)
- Breakfast bowl with ground meat, fried egg, and sautéed vegetables
- Warm quinoa with grass-fed butter and a tbsp of peanut butter (V.)
- Warm quinoa with fried eggs and greens (V.)
- Avocado toast with fried egg and salmon
- Sourdough toast topped with ricotta or cream cheese, figs or berries, and a drizzle of honey

- Mini-egg bites (see the recipe in the portal) (can also get these at the store) (V.)
- Protein pancakes (see recipe in the portal) (V.)
- Breakfast wrap: eggs and vegetables in a wrap (V.)

SUGAR-CRAVING QUICK SNACKS

Below is a list of snacks when I really need a quick handful, a good crunch, and a little pick me up while traveling, or when I am running out the door.

- Fresh berries and a handful of nuts (and chocolate chips!)
- Cut vegetables or snap peas with hummus
- Apples and nut butter with honey
- Cheese slices and apple
- Potato Chips cooked in avocado oil, olive oil, or coconut oil
- Grain-free tortilla chips cooked in avocado oil
- Meat sticks
- Raw or dry roasted nuts
- Dark chocolate chunks mixed with cashews or macadamia nuts and berries
- Whole food bars made with dried fruit and nuts
- Popcorn made with olive oil or coconut oil
- Whole milk yogurt or coconut yogurt and grain-free granola

Now let's take a quick look at what we have covered so far.

Quick Look: Committing to Your Health and Shaking Sugar

- Reflect on what it means to you to commit to your health.
- Replace refined sugar and alcohol for one week.
- Avoid artificial sweeteners found in diet drinks and foods labeled as sugar-free, such as aspartame, acesulfame potassium, saccharin, and sucralose.
- Include low-glycemic fruits and berries.
- Include protein and healthy fat at every meal, especially breakfast.
- Visit the portal for a tapping exercise on balancing blood sugar.

Disclaimer: If you feel you are experiencing an eating disorder or alcohol dependency, you may need to seek professional help from a doctor or health practitioner. Support groups like AA have also been helpful to some of my clients.

Now, we will explore the second affirmation for mood, *I respect the rhythm of my body.*

THINK: *I respect the rhythm of my body.*

Respecting your natural rhythm starts with prioritizing sleep, the foundation of your body's ability to repair, regulate, and thrive. When sleep is disrupted—whether by irregular bedtimes, artificial light exposure, or chronic stress—it throws off essential processes like metabolism, hormone regulation, and mood stability. Your body relies on deep, restful sleep. Without it, you may wake up feeling sluggish, moody, and may even struggle with cravings and weight fluctuations. Many people push past their natural cues for rest, relying on caffeine or sheer willpower to function, only to find themselves caught in a cycle of exhaustion and poor decision-making. Prioritizing a steady sleep schedule, limiting screen time before bed, and allowing your body to ease into relaxation can make all the difference in how you feel and function throughout the day.

When sleep is compromised, other natural rhythms—like digestion and energy balance—also suffer. One way this manifests is in disordered eating patterns, including skipping meals, eating at inconsistent times, or fasting without listening to the body's true needs. Your body craves stability, and when you begin to align with its natural cues—honoring rest, eating in sync with your energy needs, and allowing for a sense of ease—you create the conditions for deep, lasting vitality.

This is where this affirmation, *I respect the rhythm of my body,* becomes powerful: *Respecting your natural rhythm is a willingness to find a sense of ease with your body's energetic ebbs and flows.* Repeating this reminds you to tune in rather than push through, to allow rest rather than override exhaustion, and to make choices that support your body's well-being rather than work against it. This affirmation serves as a gentle guide, helping you reduce stress, reconnect with your intuition, and align with the natural cycles that sustain your energy. It's not just about sleep or eating habits—it's about embracing a way of living that fosters balance, renewal, and a deeper connection to yourself.

To overcome the limitations of your thoughts and personal history with dieting, use the space provided to reflect on what this affirmation means to you.

I respect the rhythm of my body.

LIVE: *Improve Sleep with PM Routines*

My Story

Many of us have an unhealthy relationship with sleep. Whether it's stealing moments of "me-time," working late, binging Netflix, or endless scrolling on our phones to avoid sleep or alleviate stress, these habits can lead to chronic sleep issues.

I remember a time when I waited for sleepiness to hit me each evening. I'd look forward to putting the kids to bed so I could watch my favorite show, which inevitably led to watching more shows, scrolling on my phone, and grabbing a snack to satiate phantom hunger cues. By the time I collapsed into bed, I'd only managed about six hours of sleep.

I thought I was a good sleeper—I usually slept through the night—but by 2 p.m. the next day, I'd feel drained, cranky, and far from my Best Energetic Self. This pattern didn't set me up for a successful evening. Dinner time became stressful and I struggled to connect with my partner and my kids before bed because I was tired and cranky. Still, I didn't want to give up my "me-time," my phone, or my shows. Those things felt like the only pieces of the day that were truly mine.

What I didn't realize then was that good sleep depends on more than just planning for eight hours. My late-night snacking taxed my liver, and the blue light from my screens overstimulated my brain, keeping it from winding down. This led to weight gain and beating myself up on the scale again. Instead of listening to my body and optimizing my sleep routine, I convinced myself that the next diet would solve everything.

Sleep Inventory

It's time to take inventory of your relationship with sleep. Write in a journal or use the space provided to reflect on the following questions:

What is your relationship with electronics or food in the evening?

_____

_____

_____

_____

How do these habits impact your sleep and mood?

_____

_____

_____

_____

What would you like to change about your relationship with sleep?

_____

_____

_____

_____

What do you think would be the first step in making that change?

_____

_____

_____

_____

How would better sleep positively impact your Best Energetic Self?

_____

_____

_____

_____

    A good night's sleep starts with a healthy evening routine. Consistently following a routine is one of the best ways to curb cravings, honor your body's internal systems, and wake up with the energy and mood to feel your best.

    One of the most common mistakes is lying in bed with a phone at night. I suggest turning off screens by 8:00 p.m. and winding down with journaling or reading by 9:00 p.m. to help induce relaxation and support your body's natural sleep rhythms. I know it's not possible for everyone to have the same schedule, so we'll customize your plan in the following section.

Sleep Deep Dive

In today's fast-paced world, we are frequently overstimulated, leaving little room to connect with ourselves. This constant state of overwhelm makes winding down feel like an insurmountable task. To cope, we often turn to food, alcohol, or TV instead of surrendering to sleep.

The benefits of quality sleep, along with a dependable evening routine, extend to every part of your body. Your sleep rhythms are crucial to tissue repair, hormone regulation, and stress processing. When you sleep well, your body thrives. When sleep is compromised, your mood and metabolism are negatively impacted. Sleep is the foundation of emotional well-being, and the lack of it can intensify negative emotions—anger, irritability, and sadness—while diminishing the positive emotions that help us feel balanced.

Unfortunately, many of us have been conditioned to see "sleepiness" as a defect. We view rest as unproductive rather than necessary. We talk about how much we need it and then resist making the changes that could resolve our sleep challenges.

We juggle responsibilities for ourselves, our families, and our work, which often leads to bedtime anxiety:

- *What didn't I finish today?*
- *What's happening tomorrow?*
- *I forgot to take care of something important.*

So, rather than succumb to sleepiness, we adopt behaviors that confuse our body's natural rhythms. These might include:

- Having another glass of wine to "relax," confusing inebriation with restfulness.

- Snacking after dinner, confusing sleepiness with hunger.
- Drinking coffee in the afternoon to push through midday tiredness, fearing a loss of productivity.
- Watching TV or scrolling on a phone, mistaking these activities for unwinding.

These habits send mixed signals to our bodies, interfering with thought patterns, eating behaviors, hormone regulation, and the energetic body.

I've had clients insist, "I have no problem sleeping—I sleep like a log!" Yet they feel tired all day, often relying on afternoon naps. You might think your sleep is fine, but if you're tired all day—even without consuming alcohol or caffeine—a poor evening ritual is likely the culprit.

It's easy to think, "TV, snacks, and phone scrolling do relax me. It's my time to unwind and enjoy what I want."

But here's the kicker: If you're still tired, moody, and frustrated with your inability to meet your health goals, then what you're currently doing is not serving you. While late-night TV, phone use, and snacks aren't inherently bad, they disrupt your body's ability to rest and recover when done right before bed. They create an unhealthy environment for your Best Energetic Self.

Many of us view sleep as a chore—something we *have* to do so we can get up to do the things we *want* to do. This mindset can turn bedtime into an anxious experience.

How often do the following thoughts occur to you?

- *I'm so tired all the time.*
- *I really need more sleep.*

- *Tonight, I won't snack after dinner. (But it happens anyway.)*
- *I'd like to stop drinking so much wine.*
- *I'm so stressed out.*

Poor sleep leaves you feeling edgy, scattered, bloated, and lethargic. Your cravings for sugar and caffeine increase, making it harder to maintain energy levels and creating a cycle of dependence on quick fixes. On top of that, sleep deprivation amplifies negative thought patterns, and this perpetuates the cycle.

The first step to better sleep is creating a shutdown routine that you love. Start by working backward from when you want to wake up, allowing at least nine or ten hours for your wind-down and sleep. This approach ensures you have time to relax and prepare for deep rest. Here's an example of an effective evening routine:

10 hours before waking up: Settle the kids or pets for the night and connect with your spouse, partner, family member, or friend. If you'd like, enjoy a short show or check social media one last time. If there are lingering tasks on your mind—like tidying the kitchen, packing lunches, folding laundry, or organizing—take care of them now so they don't weigh on you later.

9.5 hours before waking up: Switch your phone to airplane mode and avoid checking it for the rest of the night. You could also set up your phone so it automatically goes on "do not disturb." Treat yourself to something comforting, like a cup of herbal or decaf tea.

9 hours before waking up: Take this time to complete your personal care routine—taking a warm bath or shower, brushing your teeth, trimming your nails, moisturizing, or anything else that takes care of your body and relaxes your mind. Slip into comfortable pajamas.

8.5 hours before waking up: Open a journal and brain-dump any thoughts about your day that might still be swirling. Write out a schedule or to-do list for tomorrow to clear your mind. At this point, you can also fill out your *Energetic Eating* Journal food log if you didn't complete it already, your "Reflection" section, and set an intention for the following day. Then write a gratitude list of five things you're thankful for about your Best Energetic Self. If you still don't feel sleepy, read a book.

8 hours before waking up: Turn off the lights and settle into bed. Practice a body scan to relax each part of your body, from head to toe. You can use a meditation app for guided visualizations or soothing sounds to help you drift into sleep.

You can find the full evening schedule, the brain-dump exercise, and a tapping exercise for sleep in the book portal. Rewrite your routine or post it where you'll see it, and keep the brain-dump example on your bedside table for easy reference.

Disclaimer: If you are experiencing severe sleep disturbances that cannot be resolved with these adjustments, please consult a healthcare professional.

Quick Look: PM Routines

- Use the affirmation: "I respect the rhythm of my body."
- Keep a journal by your bed for brain-dumping.
- Follow the PM routine and try at least one part of the brain-dump protocol.
- Visit the book portal for a tapping exercise for better sleep.

The Power of Conscious Choices for your Mood

After years of relying on fad diets to lose weight, I finally chose to listen to my body. I committed to my health, quit drinking, and respected the rhythm of my body by replacing my evening eating rituals with rest rituals. I was able to balance my mood and transform my daily life. I went from often feeling angry and annoyed with my kids and work responsibilities to becoming more understanding and productive. I stopped loathing the person I saw in the mirror, and I had more grace with myself.

Today I savor eating a piece of dark chocolate when I am working. I grab a piece of candy from the jar at the front counter after I treat myself to a massage. I go to the local bakery for a slice of banana bread every few weeks with a friend. I occasionally binge watch my favorite shows in the evening with my partner. But I do this in alignment with my Best Energetic Self—with intentionality, reminding myself that the most important parts of who I want to be include these things in moderation, only to the extent that my mood doesn't suffer. If it does, I get to make conscious choices about sugar and sleep to turn it around.

One of my clients came to me believing her weight struggles were purely about *what* she ate—she thought the problem was simple: calories in, calories out. But it wasn't until she looked deeper that she realized it wasn't just about food—it was *how* she was living that was holding her back. She didn't have a clear reason to make changes, and she didn't understand where her cravings were coming from.

She felt trapped by her emotions, short-fused with her kids, groggy during the day, and frustrated by her inability to settle down and sleep at night. What she didn't realize was how much her nightly wine habit was disrupting her mood and her rest, keeping her stuck in a cycle of fatigue and frustration.

The breakthrough came when she replaced her evening wine with a soothing after-dinner ritual—a mocktail made with apple cider vinegar, honey, and seltzer. She followed this with a bedtime routine that included herbal tea, allowing her body to wind down naturally. Slowly, her cravings began to fade because she was finally addressing their root cause.

The transformation was powerful: fewer energy crashes, more compassion for herself and her family, and a noticeable increase in productivity at work. She no longer felt weighed down by frustration and fatigue. Instead, she gained clarity, energy, and the ability to show up for herself and her loved ones with presence and intention.

The power of these changes wasn't just in cutting out a habit—it was in recognizing that true nourishment goes beyond food. It's about understanding what your body is asking for, honoring those needs, and creating routines that support your emotional and physical well-being.

I encourage you to stick with these changes. I promise you'll see results.

When you first start incorporating these affirmations, routines, and rituals, you may feel some resistance. Most people don't want to give up their current habits, even when they leave them feeling drained or in a bad mood. In my *Energetic Eating* program, we explore the obstacles that get in the way of shaking sugar and improving sleep—time constraints, family or social commitments, and ingrained habits—and we share strategies for overcoming them.

One powerful way to stay true to your intentions is to ask yourself: What would my Best Energetic Self want me to do? This is the foundation of making conscious choices for your mood. It's about dropping habits that don't serve you, and choosing ones that do. Here's what that looks like:

- Recognizing your emotional state before making a choice. Instead of defaulting to sugar when you're low or forcing yourself to sleep at a set time when you're restless, pause. Ask yourself: What do I need right now? Sometimes it's nourishment; sometimes it's simply rest.
- Understanding that there's a time to indulge and a time to hold boundaries. Some moments call for joyful indulgence—the shared dessert on a special night, the hot cocoa on a cozy winter evening. Others require self-honoring boundaries—recognizing that sugar will deplete your energy or leave you feeling unwell. The key is making the choice from empowerment, not impulse.
- Allowing sleep to be supportive, not restrictive. A routine can be helpful but not rigid. Some nights, sleep is deep and restorative. Other nights, life happens—a late conversation, a moment of inspiration, a child who needs you. When you

trust your body, you know you'll get the rest you need without forcing it.

I know it's okay to indulge in sugar when it's part of a joyful connection rather than emotional numbing and when it's a conscious choice that won't disrupt how I want to feel later. I also know it's okay to let go of a strict sleep routine when alignment with my Best Energetic Self is worth the extra waking hours. Skipping one night of "perfect" sleep doesn't define your health.

Use the *Energetic Eating* journaling exercise below to explore how addressing committing to your health, respecting the rhythm of your body, balancing blood sugar, and improving sleep can benefit you. The journal includes prompts to help if you're feeling stuck.

This is the real shift—from rules to self-trust, from restriction to alignment, from reacting to choosing. Every day is a new opportunity to listen, honor, and decide what serves you best.

Date: _____

MIT(s): *What is the most important thing you'd like to focus on from your Best Energetic Self?*		
How I Think:	How I Eat:	How I Live:
What is a positive thought or affirmation that you would like to take with you?	*When you think about supporting yourself nutritionally, what could that look like now?*	*When you think about supporting yourself through lifestyle choices, what could that look like now?*

Breakfast: How did you feel?	
Lunch: How did you feel?	
Dinner: How did you feel?	
Snack 1: How did you feel?	Snack 2: How did you feel?
Liquids: How did you feel?	
Reflection: *How are you feeling today? How has making these shifts positively influenced your Best Energetic Self?*	

CHAPTER 6

PILLAR 3: YOUR DIGESTION

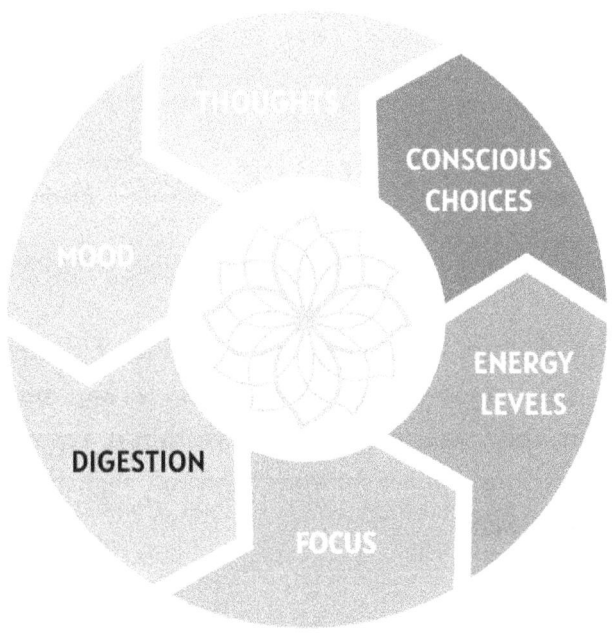

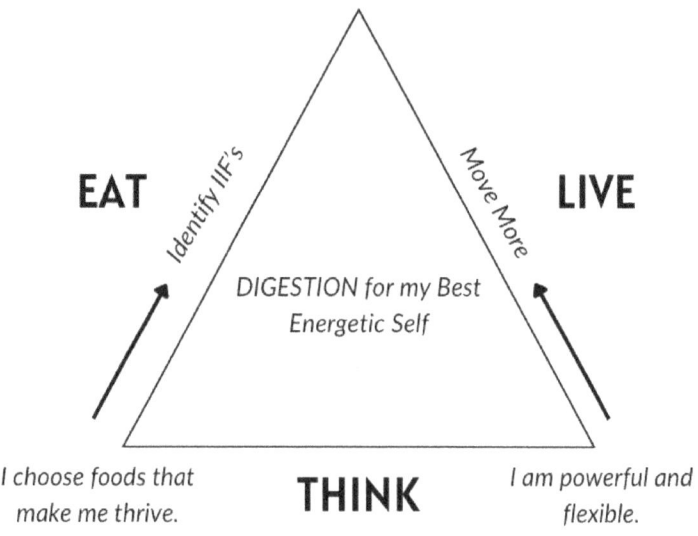

In this chapter, we will explore the Think, Eat, Live Triad through two empowering affirmations, a key nutritional component, and a transformative lifestyle shift to support you in making conscious choices for your digestion aligned with your Best Energetic Self.

Overview

The digestive system is responsible for delivering nutrients to every part of your body, and how your digestion feels is a major factor in supporting your Best Energetic Self. At the height of my yo-yo dieting, I dealt with poor digestion: reflux, gas, and bloating. I was even diagnosed with IBS—a clear sign that something was out of balance. But instead of heeding the signals and understanding how to heal this inflammatory stress, I continued to focus my energy on fad weight-loss tricks.

Digestion isn't just about gas, bloating, and bowel movements. Did you know that 90% of your serotonin—a neurotransmitter crucial for regulating mood, sleep, and appetite—is made in the gut? Poor digestion can do more than cause discomfort; it can lead to brain fog, depression, anxiety, cravings, and disordered eating patterns like overeating or undereating. It can also manifest in unexpected ways, contributing to issues like eczema, joint pain, and chronic inflammation. Your gut health influences far more than digestion—it impacts your entire body and mind. In this chapter, we'll address the mindset tools to support digestion in the "Think" sections. Each affirmation will also include an "Eat" or "Live" component to help you heal digestive issues.

Digestion Foods Reflection

Rate each of the following on a scale of 1–5, with 1 meaning "never," 3 meaning "sometimes," and 5 meaning "always." Consider these questions in relation to the past six months.

- Do you get heartburn or acid reflux?
- Do you have constipation or diarrhea?
- Do you struggle with anxious thoughts and feelings?
- Do you feel foggy midday?
- Do you have uncomfortable and embarrassing gas?

Total: ___ out of 25

If you scored 15 or higher, the suggestions in this chapter will be especially helpful for you to explore and implement.

Now, let's explore the affirmations, nutrition, and lifestyle strategies that will support your digestion.

THINK: *I choose foods that make me thrive.*

The key takeaway about choosing foods (or drinks) that help you thrive is that the right choice for you doesn't always align with the "healthy" diet standard. When I followed a vegan diet, I ate what was considered super healthy—soy products, grains, cereal products, black bean burgers, and fake meats. While these foods might work well for others, they didn't let me thrive, and in fact, my heavy reliance on them left me in extreme digestive distress.

What I didn't realize was that I had a sensitivity to lectins and legumes, which triggered an inflammatory response in my digestive system. I couldn't eat anything without experiencing gas and bloating. Choosing foods that help us thrive starts with understanding how different foods affect us, enabling us to make conscious choices to feel good. Some foods can become non-negotiable for you because you are allergic or they make you feel so terrible that avoiding them is the right choice. Examples might include lactose for those with intolerance or gluten for those with celiac disease. Other foods might work in moderation. For instance, I've found that a slice or two of sourdough bread per week is fine for me, but eating it daily leaves me feeling foggy and anxious. Pizza once a month is manageable, but ordering and eating take out for a few days in a row leaves me sluggish and digestively unwell. This is the energy of food in my body. Listening closely is the key.

Every person has a unique set of "individual inflammatory foods" (and some people have none at all). In addition to listening to inflammatory responses in the body, it's also important to connect your food and drink choices with your Best Energetic Self. A glass of wine while catching up with an old friend feels different than having one every night. Ordering a kid-sized cup of ice cream is different from indulging in a jumbo cone. Indulging in high-quality dark chocolate is different from giving yourself permission to eat all of the candy because it is Halloween. We know this based on how we feel.

If your food and drink choices seem to get in the way of you feeling digestively well, it's time to reassess. Use the resources provided in this chapter to pinpoint the problem areas without relying on what you think you know from fad diets.

To overcome the limitations of your thoughts and personal history with dieting, use the space provided to reflect on what this affirmation means to you.

I choose foods that make me thrive.

EAT: *Individual Inflammatory Foods*

My Story

For me, digestion was my number one frustration throughout my 20s. I had such intense bloating and discomfort that I often called in late to work or canceled plans. I even left a date early because I was so worried about my gas!

During this time, my diet revolved around keeping my food points low. I'd start the day with a fat-free yogurt and high-fiber muffin, followed by a soy milk latte for lunch and a bean or legume-based dinner. To cope with the resulting weight gain, gas, and constipation, I turned to week-long juice fasts, raw fruit and vegetable diets, laxative teas, and enemas. While these often gave me temporary relief, the same discomfort returned the moment I resumed eating normally.

Proper digestion gives you increased energy, self-confidence, and comfort. When your body's natural processes are functioning well, your belly feels supple. You burp infrequently, your bowel movements are regular and complete, gas is minimal, and reflux is often resolved. When your body feels this way, you are effectively assimilating nutrients to keep you healthy and energized, directly supporting your Best Energetic Self.

When I was dealing with digestive issues, I lacked energy and confidence. The food choices I sought comfort in made me feel worse. I joined a weight-loss support program to manage my weight, but the points system kept me focused on weight loss rather than the nutrients and digestion it needed to thrive.

Your journey cannot be about weight loss alone. You have to become invested in *feeling good* and commit to identifying the foods that make you feel bad—not just those that you believe will help you lose weight. Low-calorie, low-fat, and low-point foods do not necessarily support digestion, even if they help you shed a few pounds. The weight will likely come back, and the cycle will begin again.

Inflammatory Foods Inventory

Inflammatory foods can cause a variety of uncomfortable symptoms and disrupt your overall well-being. Take a moment now to take inventory of your relationship with inflammatory foods. Write in a journal or use the space provided to reflect on the following questions:

How often do you feel digestively unwell (gas, bloating, abdominal pain, inconsistent or infrequent bowel movements)?

_____
_____
_____
_____

How does poor digestion impact how you feel about your body?

_____
_____
_____
_____

What would you like to change about your relationship with foods that cause digestive disturbances?

_____
_____
_____
_____

What do you think would be the first step in making that change?

_____

_____

_____

_____

How would these changes positively impact your Best Energetic Self?

_____

_____

_____

_____

Once I evaluated my relationship with inflammatory foods and began to make changes, I discovered that feeling good in my body mattered more than sticking with a diet. Identifying and addressing my individual inflammatory foods significantly improved my digestion and overall quality of life.

Individual Inflammatory Foods Deep Dive

Everyone has a unique set of individual inflammatory foods ("IIFs"), but there are common foods to which many people develop sensitivities due to highly processed ingredients, overconsumption, and stress. To uncover your IIFs, you'll need to investigate which foods are safe for you, which are tolerable in moderation, and which are non-negotiable based on how you feel after eating them.

When digestion is out of balance, many of us fall into a "screw it" mentality—giving in to impulse, eating whatever we want, and experiencing negative symptoms or weight gain, only to dig around for another diet in the name of weight loss. But I want you to let it matter more.

When your body digests food properly, it balances blood sugar, assimilates nutrients, and moves waste efficiently through the large intestine. Many of my clients who experience digestive issues find relief by addressing common inflammatory foods, such as sugar and alcohol (which we have already covered), gluten, grains, dairy, soy products, gums, and thickening agents in processed food. Addressing these issues starts with listening to your body and recognizing the symptoms it's signaling. Some of my clients have discovered that their digestive issues stem from less commonly recognized inflammatory foods, such as high-fat meats, nightshades, or beans and legumes.

If you take a week-long break from sugar and alcohol, as we discussed in Chapter 5, and don't find complete digestive relief, the next step is to remove gluten for a week, then grains the next. These elements—sugar, alcohol, gluten, and grains—can create an inflammatory "wall" that masks what's truly triggering your symptoms. By removing them one at a time, you allow potential inflammatory triggers to "speak more loudly," making it easier to identify if other foods could be affecting you. This process clears the path to uncovering the root cause of your discomfort.

During this process, I guide my clients to evaluate the effects other foods have on their bodies by journaling—not about quantities or macros, but about how they feel after eating. Notes like *I feel overly full*, *I feel bloated*, or *I feel sick to my stomach* provide valuable clues without feeding into the obsessive tendencies driven by fad dieting. (Remember, this is about how you feel, not about weight loss.) Once relief is found, you can reintroduce foods one at a time in reverse order—starting with grains, then gluten, and finally sugar (say, twice a week)—paying attention to how your body responds to each, without overwhelming your system. This step-by-step process allows you to peel back the layers, gain clarity, use the insights from your journaling to investigate and address the way you feel for your Best Energetic Self, and learn how to eat foods in moderation.

You can read the tables below and visit the book portal for a comprehensive list of potentially inflammatory foods and suggestions for swaps that may work better for you. I have also included acupressure for digestive relief after eating in the portal.

Here's a table of common symptoms from common foods linked to potential IIFs, and suggested swaps to help you feel your best. They are in order of how I guide my clients to explore the impact of their individual inflammatory foods. Use this as a guide to start identifying patterns and making conscious choices for better digestion.

\multicolumn{3}{c}{**GLUTEN, GRAINS, & GUMS**}		
Symptoms	Gluten/ Grain/ Gums	SWAP
Energy crash, food addiction, headaches, stubborn weight, acid reflux, eczema, fatigue, mood swings	Pastries Or Muffins	Limit, replace with protein-based breakfasts from Chapter 5, and try making muffins that swap flour for almond flour and sugar for honey
Diarrhea, constipation, fatigue, headaches, eczema, stubborn weight, acid reflux	Bread	Roasted potatoes, sweet potato buns, collard green wraps, coconut wraps, and fresh sourdough bread can be tolerated by many individuals
Coughing, indigestion, gas, bloating, fatigue, stubborn weight, food addiction	Corn & Hidden Corn • Dextri-maltose • Dextrin • Dextrose • Fructose • Glucose and glucose Syrup • Cereal starch • Modified starch • High fructose corn syrup	→ Grain-free almond or cassava tortillas, grain-free tortilla chips, cauliflower or egg wraps

ENERGETIC EATING | 121

GLUTEN, GRAINS, & GUMS		
Symptoms	Gluten/ Grain/ Gums	SWAP
Same as bread and pastries	Pizza	→ Cauliflower crust or almond flour crust
Indigestion, mood swings, gas, diarrhea or constipation, cravings for sweets or alcohol, depression, fatigue	Yeast Sugar, Fermented, And High Carbohydrate-Containing Foods, Alcohol Most Gluten-Containing Foods High Carbohydrate Fruit: Bananas, Plums, Prunes, Figs, Dates, Raisins, Grapes	Low added sugar and carbohydrates; reduce alcohol from daily to twice weekly; some may have to eliminate it Cut bread from four slices a day to two and pasta from four days to two days a week can help Berries, melons, an apple or grapefruit
Diarrhea, constipation, fatigue, headaches, nausea, mood swings, stubborn weight, reflux	Rice, Brown Rice, Oats (less common)	Recipes with wild rice, quinoa, cauliflower rice, millet

| Gas, bloating, constipation, stomach pain, diarrhea | Gums and thickeners in many gluten-free and dairy-free products (carrageenan, xanthan gum, gum acacia, food starches, such as potato, tapioca, and cornstarch). found in packaged "gluten-free" foods, powders, mixes, and dairy alternatives. | Read your food labels, choose fresh when possible, and make delicious gluten-free goods made from cassava or nut flours. |

OTHER LESS COMMON IIFs

Explore these foods in order if you don't have relief from the common IIFs

Symptoms	IIFs	→	Swap
Gastrointestinal distress such as gas, bloating, cramps, constipation	Soybean oil, vegetable oil, soy sauce	→	Olive oil (low-medium heat) or avocado oil (high heat), coconut aminos
Stomach pain, one-sided headaches, constipation, sleepy after eating fats	High-fat foods (fried foods, fatty meats)	→	Pasture-raised, lean meats and fish, lentils, steamed or sautéed vegetables fry/bake in avocado oil
Abdominal pain, bloating, diarrhea, gas, nausea, breakouts, restlessness, irritability, difficulty sleeping	Dairy	→	Canned coconut milk without added guar gum, oat, almond, or cashew milk without added gums or sugar. You can sub dairy cheese with avocado or nut cheese.

Bloating, gas, abdominal cramps, thyroid issues	Lectins/ legumes, i.e.: Beans, chickpea, lentil, soybean	→	Cashew cheese, cauliflower hummus, cook beans with ginger and bay leaf, or use ground meat, shredded chicken, or try taking a digestive enzyme before your meal
Achy muscles or joints, skin issues, rosacea, psoriasis	Nightshades: tomatoes, peppers, chilies, eggplant, potatoes	→	Remove the skin; if still symptomatic, avoid these foods

Many of my clients feel anxious about upcoming events or celebrations when evaluating IIFs. If this resonates with you, ask yourself a few guiding questions:

- Will this food cause extreme digestive issues or stress on my body?
- Are there alternatives I can choose instead?
- Can I indulge in an appetizer portion or stick to a palm-sized serving?
- Can I eat half and feel satisfied?

The good news is that most people can limit inflammatory foods, improve digestion, and reintroduce them in moderation. The key is in how you feel.

Let's address the gluten-free hype. Unfortunately, as gluten-free has become a popular marketing ploy, many processed gluten-free foods are filled with added starches and gums—like modified food starch, xanthan gum, and guar gum—that can wreak havoc on the gut and digestion. Unless you have sensitivities to grains, when choosing gluten-free options, look for ones made with oats, brown rice, white rice, or quinoa without those added ingredients. If you are sensitive to grains, choose options made with nut flours. Be mindful that corn, often found in gluten-free pasta and other products, can also cause digestive issues for many people.

It's best to prioritize minimally processed food like pasture-raised meat, fish, eggs, fruits, and vegetables. Rather than pairing these with gluten, have a vegetable instead. Some examples:

- Replace a sandwich with a lettuce wrap or a salad topped with your favorite sandwich fillings.
- Serve eggs on roasted potatoes instead of toast.
- Snack on cassava chips, vegetables, guacamole, cheese, nut butter, apples, or fruit. If you stop feeling undesirable symptoms once you eliminate gluten, you can reintroduce options like sourdough bread (which contains less gluten and yeast).
- Try quinoa, millet, and rice and see how your body feels.

In addition to limiting foods that cause inflammation, you can focus on foods that actively reduce it. Vegetables, low-glycemic fruits, prebiotics, and probiotics can effectively improve digestion and overall health. Simply ensuring that you eat six cups of varied, colorful veggies maximizes fiber intake, enhancing your digestion and giving you the essential nutrients you could be lacking, helping you feel better immediately.

Fiber is essential for a healthy digestive system. It helps:

- Regulate bowel movements.
- Prevent constipation.
- Promote the growth of healthy gut bacteria.
- Slow sugar absorption to balance blood sugar.
- Increase feelings of fullness and reduce cravings.

Vegetables are rich in soluble and insoluble fiber. Soluble fiber absorbs and forms a gel-like substance in your gut, aiding digestion, while insoluble fiber adds bulk to your stool, promoting regularity. Eating a variety of vegetables, such as cruciferous veggies (like kale and Brussels sprouts), leafy greens, and colorful options, ensures you get a balance of both types of fiber, which are crucial for your overall gut health.

Two of your six cups can come from low-glycemic fruits, like strawberries, raspberries, blueberries, apples, pears, and cherries. These fruits are packed with fiber, antioxidants, and vitamins that support overall health while keeping blood sugar levels stable. You don't need to count or measure—six cups means that you focus on including them often, even as a part of every meal.

To further support digestion, incorporate foods that nourish your gut microbiome.

- Probiotic foods: These contain live beneficial bacteria that help balance the microorganisms in your digestive system and introduce "good" bacteria that aid digestion and improve nutrient absorption. Examples include fermented foods like yogurt, kefir, sauerkraut, kimchi, miso, and kombucha.

- Prebiotic foods: These feed the beneficial bacteria in your gut and enhance your ability to produce short-chain fatty acids that support digestion. Great prebiotic options include garlic, onions, leeks, asparagus, and artichokes.

Visit the book portal for a printable table with a comprehensive list of foods that support digestion and inflammation reduction, which you can also find in the table provided.

SUPPORT YOUR DIGESTION	
Type	Examples
Fiber- rich foods	Broccoli, kale, Brussels sprouts, spinach, carrots, celery, bell peppers
Low-glycemic fruits	Berries (strawberries, raspberries, blueberries), apples, pears, cherries
Probiotic foods	Yogurt, kefir, sauerkraut, kimchi, miso, kombucha
Prebiotic foods	Garlic, onions, leeks, asparagus, artichokes

Disclaimer: Seek help from doctors if you are experiencing serious digestive issues or food allergies.

Quick Look: Choosing Foods That Make You Thrive and IIFs

- Reflect on what it means to choose foods that make you thrive.
- To identify your IIFs, keep a daily log for the next week, remembering first to eliminate sugar and alcohol, then common gluten and grains, and then the other IIFs if necessary. Be curious about how foods affect you, then reintroduce them as outlined in this chapter. You can use the *Energetic Eating* journal format or print an example from the portal to help record how you feel.
- Include six cups of vegetables (and low-glycemic fruits), prebiotics, and probiotics.
- Acupressure points for digestive relief are demonstrated in the book portal.

Now, we will explore the second affirmation of digestion.

THINK: *I am powerful and flexible.*

Being powerful and flexible is the opposite of an all-or-nothing mindset—true power comes from flexibility in our thinking and choices. Instead of creating rigid rules, we can explore what is possible, allowing ourselves to adapt to life's changes, our evolving needs, and the unexpected challenges that inevitably arise. For example, many people believe they must set the bar high and reach it or maintain continuous improvement, or else they are failures. You might think, "If I ran two miles yesterday, I must do the same or better today," or, "I'm too tired today, so I'll skip it entirely." This very common rigid thinking protects us from disappointment, but stands in the way of our progress.

But what if our true power and potential lie in meeting ourselves where we are? If we believed that were true, we'd be able to say, "I ran two miles yesterday. I wonder how far my body will go today?" or "Even though I feel tired, I can still move in a way that feels good." Talking to yourself this way will help you learn to move through resistance.

This applies in any situation. How often do you back down from something because it feels hard, and what would it be like not to take on the entire challenge but just a piece of it? And when it comes to food, instead of saying, "screw it" and eating the whole thing, ask yourself, "What are my options?" and know that you can have less, stop midway, or choose a better alternative.

Fad diets tell us that power comes from rigidly following the rules. The truth is, power comes from deciding among the variety of options available to us and meeting yourself where you are.

To overcome the limitations of your thoughts and personal history with dieting, use the space provided to reflect on what this affirmation means to you.

I am powerful and flexible.

LIVE: *Increase Movement*

My Story

I've had an on-again, off-again relationship with movement. For years, it was tied to one goal: losing weight. Every effort felt like a sprint toward a finish line—whether it was signing up for marathon training, diving into a 90-day challenge, or pushing myself through the latest intense workout trend. But that all-or-nothing approach was never sustainable. It wasn't about listening to my body; it was about pushing through, no matter the cost. And the cost? It was high. Not only did I burn out, but I also ended up hurting myself along the way.

After having my second child, I felt that familiar urgency to "bounce back" and shed the baby weight. Six weeks after giving birth, I laced up my shoes and went for a run—determined, but not truly ready. Almost immediately, I felt it: pain in my hips and knees, something I had never experienced before. It was a wake-up call, forcing me to face a hard truth—I couldn't just force my body back into movement the way I used to. Something had to change.

This time, instead of focusing on the weight, I focused on the pain. I asked myself, *What does my body need to feel supported, strong, and whole again?* That question led me to a postpartum Pilates class, where the focus was on rebuilding, not shrinking. I also began a gentle walk/run-to-5K program that taught me the power of starting small. I learned how to slow down to truly move forward—how to honor where I was instead of fighting against it. Slowing down and listening to my body wasn't a setback—it was where real progress happened.

Movement Inventory

Let's take a moment to take inventory of your relationship with movement. Write in a journal or use the space provided to reflect on the following questions:

How often do you choose sedentary tasks (i.e., phone scrolling, binge-watching television) over moving your body?

_____

_____

_____

_____

How does digestion impact your desire to move?

_____

_____

_____

_____

What would you like to change about your relationship with movement?

_____

_____

_____

_____

What do you think would be the first step in making that change?

_____

_____

_____

_____

How would these changes positively impact your Best Energetic Self?

_____

_____

_____

_____

Movement Deep Dive

Regular movement plays a crucial role in supporting digestion by enhancing the natural processes of the gastrointestinal system and promoting overall gut health. Physical activity stimulates intestinal muscle contractions, known as peristalsis, which helps food and waste move efficiently through the digestive tract, reducing bloating and preventing constipation. Exercise also improves blood flow to the digestive organs, enhancing their ability to break down food and absorb nutrients. Additionally, movement lowers stress levels by reducing cortisol, which is particularly important since stress can negatively impact digestion by slowing motility or causing inflammation. Regular activity also promotes a healthier balance of gut bacteria, which are essential for digestion, immunity, and overall health.

Furthermore, movement activates the lymphatic system, aiding in the removal of toxins and waste that can otherwise burden the digestive system. Even light activity, such as a gentle walk after a meal, can kick-start digestion and reduce common discomforts like heartburn or bloating. Incorporating regular physical activity into your daily routine is a simple yet effective way to support digestion and improve overall well-being.

One solution that works for my clients is to start gently with walking/speed-walking or walking/jogging intervals, gradually increasing active time while reducing rest intervals. For example, 60 seconds jogging or speed-walking and 90 seconds walking for one or two miles 2–3 times per week.

Interval training can help you meet yourself where you are instead of pushing you beyond your limits, leading to burnout. If you are curious, explore apps that support walk/run interval training or check out my *Energetic Way to 5k* guide, complete with intervals and affirmations, in the book portal.

Strength training is another powerful way to boost your body's energy and resilience. It's not just about building physical strength—it's about activating your energy, fostering resilience, and creating a foundation for vibrant health. When I work with my clients, I suggest starting twice per week. They progress from gentle, intentional movements to more dynamic weight training, always focusing on aligning the body's strength with its natural energy flow, without pushing past pain or physical discomfort. By engaging in strength training, you're tapping into the deeper layers of health—balancing your physical body with the subtle energy systems that support it. As muscles strengthen and energy builds, you'll feel an unmistakable shift: you'll become more grounded, empowered, and connected to your body. This practice is not about forcing change, but about aligning with the inherent strength and vitality already within you. Progression is key. You can find examples of workout progressions in the book portal.

Yoga has become a grounding ritual in my workout routine, one that I turn to, not for hours of effort, but for its simplicity, accessibility, and powerful effects on my energy and well-being. Choosing online yoga sessions that are 20 minutes or less allows me to weave this practice into my day when I feel like I have very little time—whether it's to find balance in the morning, reset during a busy afternoon, or unwind before bed.

Here are some other simple yet effective ways to commit to more movement:

- Stand instead of sitting when possible (e.g., at your desk, on phone calls).
- Use a treadmill designed to go in front of your desk to walk while working.
- Park a little farther away and walk more.
- Take the stairs instead of the elevator.
- Challenge yourself to walk when you go anywhere that's less than two miles away. Do it in *any* weather (safety permitting, of course).
- Take walking meetings or walk daily at lunchtime. Do it outside if you can.
- Sit on the floor while watching TV to engage your core. You might even feel inspired to do a little stretching or some core exercises.

- Use apps or calendar events to remind you to stretch and move.
- Wear sneakers and/or dress in your workout clothes to inspire extra movement.
- Use a foam roller to reduce stress and move lymph in your body. You can find YouTube videos to help you.
- Join your kids or pets for 10 minutes of fun when they run around the house or play sports.

A printable list is available in the book portal.

Humans are made to move. Exercise is necessary for a long and healthy life and for cultivating the belief that you can push through hard things mentally. While hiring a personal trainer can provide valuable guidance, it can be expensive. Signing up for a class might seem like a great option, but it can also feel intimidating, and some women worry that the activity will be too difficult or they're anxious about how they look. These concerns often lead us to put off movement, telling ourselves we'll start "when the time is right." But here's the truth: the mental resistance you feel—whether it's about lack of time, self-consciousness, cost, or any other excuses—is your sign to move. The "right time" is now, and the most effective way to move through this resistance is accountability.

That's why I recommend the "swim buddy" approach, a principle from Navy SEAL training. In training camp, each person is assigned a swim buddy—a partner who is responsible for supporting them through every challenge. This partnership is about more than just accountability; it's about survival.

The key to a successful swim buddy partnership is finding someone who is equally as invested in your well-being as you are.

This can't be someone who will be your buddy in skipping workouts to watch a show instead. You have to be invested in mutual well-being.

Here are some swim buddy ideas:

The Check-in System – Set up a daily or weekly check-in with your swim buddy. This could be a quick text, a voice note, or a five-minute call to share your wins, challenges, and next steps. The goal is to keep each other engaged, not just accountable.

Parallel Progress – Even if you're not doing the exact same workout, commit to making progress together. One person might be focusing on strength training while the other is working on running—but you're both committed to growth and can celebrate each other's progress.

SOS Support – When motivation dips or obstacles arise, a swim buddy is the person you call before giving up. If you're struggling to stick to a commitment, instead of ghosting your plan, you reach out, get encouragement, and find a way forward together.

The Commitment Contract – Write down your goals together and create a simple agreement—what you both want to achieve, how you'll support each other, and what happens if one of you falls off track. Knowing you have a shared pact strengthens follow-through.

Active Buddying – If possible, work out together, take walks while catching up, or go to a class together. This makes the process social and enjoyable rather than feeling like a solo grind.

Disclaimer: If you are experiencing extreme fatigue where you cannot increase movement without exhaustion or pain, please see a healthcare professional.

Quick Look: Power and Flexibility and Movement

- Reflect on what it means to be powerful and flexible.
- Choose three movements from the list to try today.
- Find a "swim buddy" for accountability.
- Visit the portal for the *Energetic Way to 5k* guide and strength training exercises.

The Power of Conscious Choices with Your Digestion

I went from struggling with extreme digestive distress to truly listening to my body and honoring what it needed. Avoiding soy products is non-negotiable for me, and while I haven't been able to adhere to a strict vegetarian diet, I can enjoy beans and legumes about once a week and gluten-containing foods about twice a week without experiencing undesirable digestive distress or other symptoms.

Over time, I also built an exercise routine that supports me, starting with small steps like completing walk/run 5K training. It has since grown to include strength training, jogging, and playing tennis and basketball. My Best Energetic Self depended on my moving more, so I naturally shifted my focus to foods that nourish me, choosing options that helped me feel well enough to move my body in the way I want to and in ways I never thought would be possible.

Had I stayed stuck in the all-or-nothing mindset—accepting digestive discomfort as normal and relying on short-term diets and die-hard exercise plans—I'd still be bloated, frustrated, and unhappy with my body. Instead, I found sustainable habits based on my IIFs and healed my digestion with prebiotic and probiotic foods. I chose exercise that met my needs, not a caloric deficit or a weight-loss goal. It was the healing that helped me trust my body and stop looking for another diet to control my weight. I know this approach can work for you, too.

One of my clients came to me hyper-focused on weight loss. She had tried nearly everything—counting points, following a low-fat diet, and restricting calories. And while each method helped her lose weight for a short period of time, the weight always came back. What she didn't realize was that her body was signaling something deeper. Alongside her struggle with weight, she was experiencing irregular bowel movements—swinging between sudden urges and complete inactivity. It had gotten so severe that she had to plan her mornings around going to the bathroom.

Desperate for answers, she visited multiple doctors, all of whom dismissed her concerns with a vague diagnosis of IBS and no clear solution. When she came to me, she was expecting another one-size-fits-all diet plan—but I asked her to do something different. For one week, she journaled not just her food intake but also her lifestyle habits and her thoughts about herself.

When we reviewed her journal together, one pattern stood out—even though she strived for a calorie deficit, gluten and sugars from processed food were a constant presence in her diet. We decided to experiment by eliminating them and seeing how her body responded. Within three days, everything changed. Her digestive issues eased, the bloating subsided, and the cravings that once felt uncontrollable began to quiet. She finally trusted her body enough in the mornings to start a walk/run routine that led her to feeling strong and capable.

But the most profound shift wasn't just physical—it was in how she saw herself. The thoughts that had weighed on her for years—believing she was a failure, broken, or destined to be "sick"—began to dissolve. As her body started to heal, her mindset transformed too. She no longer viewed herself through the lens of defeat but through a growing sense of confidence and well-being. After a week, she slowly incorporated small amounts of gluten and enjoyed less-processed sweet snacks without disrupting her digestion again. Connecting her body with the way she felt was crucial in helping her stay consistent for the long term.

I've seen this transformation happen for many of my clients. Sometimes it's gluten; sometimes it's another seemingly harmless food like beans. The real breakthrough happens when you become your own detective, tuning into your body through the symptoms you are experiencing.

The lesson here is about understanding what you're thinking about yourself, how different foods make you feel, and the lifestyle choices you are making for your Best Energetic Self. When you start paying attention to your body's signals and honoring what it needs, that's when true healing and transformation begin.

When you first start incorporating these affirmations, habits, routines, and rituals, you may feel some resistance. Most people feel resistant to giving up their current eating rituals, even when these habits leave them feeling digestively sluggish or uncomfortable. In the *Energetic Eating Method*, I review food journals to compassionately help clients discover the foods that work for them. You might benefit from working with a coach, dietitian, or nutritionist, but be sure to choose someone who helps you understand yourself deeply—and more comprehensively than as just a product of the foods you eat or a number on the scale.

Remember to ask yourself: What would my Best Energetic Self want me to do?

This is the foundation of making conscious choices for your digestion. It's about choosing food from a place of empowerment rather than impulse, and choosing exercise that feels good. Here's what that looks like:

- Recognizing how food makes you feel before making a choice. Instead of blindly following a list of "good" or "bad" foods, tune in. Ask yourself: How does this food support me? Do I feel energized, light, and nourished after eating it, or heavy and sluggish? Not every day will be the same, and that's okay.
- Understanding there's a time to be mindful of individual inflammatory foods and a time to simply enjoy life. Some moments call for choosing the foods that fuel digestion and movement, while others call for letting go of rigidity and trusting your body's resilience. When you make choices from a place of empowerment rather than fear, food

becomes something that supports your body instead of something to control.
- Allowing movement to be supportive, not punishing. Movement is not just about burning calories or "making up" for food choices—it's about creating energy, supporting digestion, and strengthening the connection between mind and body. Instead of forcing workouts that feel like punishment, choose movement that feels like self-care and aligns with your Best Energetic Self.

I know it's fine to enjoy a food that might not be "perfect" for digestion when I'm fully present with the experience and not eating out of guilt or habit. I also know it's okay to rest when my body needs it, without fear of losing progress. Skipping one day of movement doesn't mean I'm failing—it means I'm listening.

Use the *Energetic Eating* journaling exercise below to explore how conscious choices can support your Best Energetic Self. You can now add "Think," "Eat," and "Live" components from this chapter. Prompts are included in the journal to guide you if you feel stuck.

This is the real shift—from rules to self-trust, from restriction to alignment, from reacting to choosing. Every day is a new opportunity to listen, honor, and decide what serves you best.

Date: _____

MIT(s): *What is the most important thing you'd like to focus on from your Best Energetic Self?*		
How I Think:	How I Eat:	How I Live:
What is a positive thought or affirmation that you would like to take with you?	*When you think about supporting yourself nutritionally, what could that look like now?*	*When you think about supporting yourself through lifestyle choices, what could that look like now?*

Breakfast: How did you feel?
Lunch: How did you feel?
Dinner: How did you feel?

Snack 1: How did you feel?	Snack 2: How did you feel?

Liquids: How did you feel?
Reflection: *How are you feeling today? How has making these shifts positively influenced your Best Energetic Self?*

CHAPTER 7

PILLAR 4: YOUR FOCUS

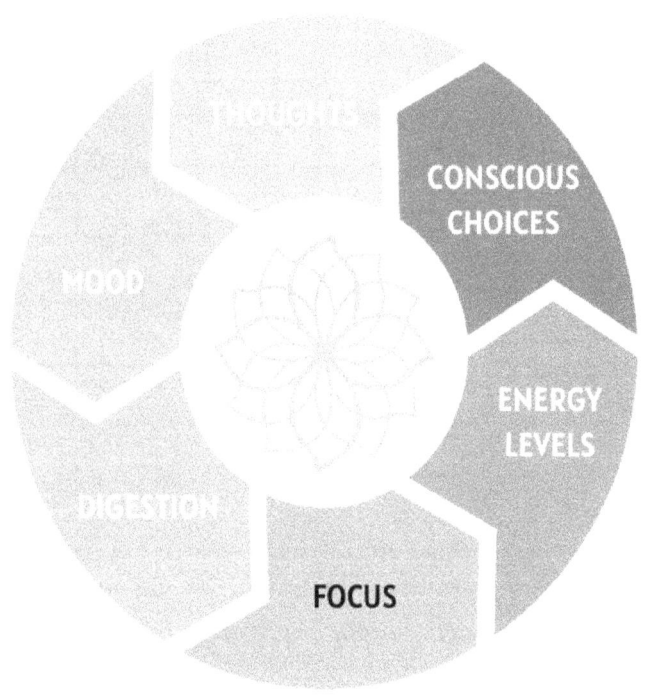

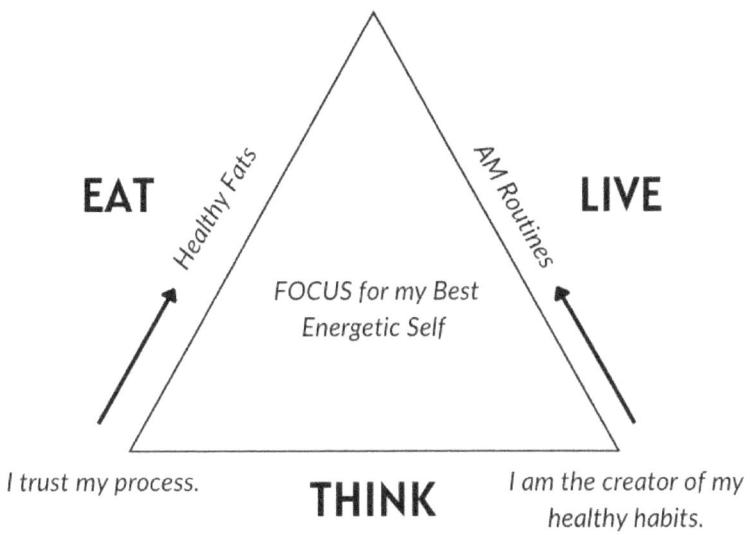

In this chapter, through the Think, Eat, Live Triad, we'll explore two empowering affirmations, a key nutritional component, and a transformative lifestyle shift to help you make conscious choices for your focus aligned with your Best Energetic Self.

Overview

This pillar focuses on a common sign of inflammation—lack of focus—which can arise from a deficiency in healthy fats that support brain function and the absence of a grounding morning practice. Lack of focus often manifests as brain fog, walking into rooms and forgetting why you're there, struggling to disengage from social media, or feeling scattered and overwhelmed.

We'll explore how the rise of convenience foods has led to overconsumption of unhealthy fats, and how crowding out unhealthy fats is essential for brain health. I'll also introduce a morning routine designed to help you start your day with clarity, intention, and a sense of well-being.

Focus Reflection

Rate each of the following on a scale of 1–5, with 1 meaning "never," 3 meaning "sometimes," and 5 meaning "always." Consider these questions in relation to the past six months.

- Do you feel scatterbrained?
- Do you get brain fog?
- Is it hard for you to stick with tasks?
- Do you use your phone when other important things need to get done?
- Do you turn to food when other important things need to get done?

Total: ___ out of 25

If you scored 15 or higher, the suggestions in this chapter will be especially helpful for you to explore and implement. Now, let's explore an affirmation that will support your ability to stay focused.

THINK: *I trust my process.*

Trusting your process helps you reframe failure as winning. Changing your eating and lifestyle behaviors takes time, and the journey can feel discouraging. When you're in the middle of a long-term adjustment or life change, your mindset becomes your greatest tool for support.

Repeating the affirmation, "I trust my process," helps you stay open to learning and growth, even when things feel challenging, difficult, or frustrating.

In the past, you may have viewed quitting as proof that you were incapable. But today, I want you to see that everything you've done, including quitting, has been necessary for you to arrive exactly where you need to be. When you see the whole picture as a part of a process rather than a race to an end goal, you become more present in your day-to-day actions. Instead of beating yourself up over your choices, you can say, "I trust my process."

Fad diets convince us that weight loss depends on strict systems of counting, measuring, and controlling food. As you'll learn in this chapter, outdated beliefs, like the obsession with low-fat and non-fat products, still fuel the diet mentality today. But the truth is, food isn't about rules; it's about alignment. Every choice either supports how you want to feel or takes you further from it.

If you tend to be anxious or regretful about your choices, take a moment to reflect. Use the provided space to write about what trusting your process means to you.

I trust my process.

Now that you've explored what it means to trust your process, let's explore the "Eat" portion of the triad as it relates to focus.

EAT: *Healthy Fats*

My Story

It was 1998, and I vividly remember being influenced by the low-fat/no-fat program commercials. I would hunt for the bright green labels on packages that signaled reduced fat, like the one on the reduced-fat cookies or the bright blue cap on a gallon of skim milk. When I went to college, the staple dorm room snack was a slice of bread sprayed with a butter-flavored vegetable oil and dusted with cinnamon sugar. It felt like we were all in on some secret formula—one that promised weight loss and health through fat-free everything.

For years, I thought fat was the enemy—a so-called "weight-gain food." I avoided it at all costs. All the commercials and diet literature led me to seek out low-fat and fat-free packaged foods, believing they were the key to staying lean. But instead of feeling energized, I found myself constantly hungry, craving more, and stuck in a cycle of overeating. My meals were filled with sugar-laden, processed substitutes for real food, and I didn't understand the impact this was having on my body. Those choices, the ones I thought were "healthy," were actually setting me back. The lack of healthy fats contributed to the food addiction, digestive issues, and brain fog that I later had to untangle.

Take a moment to reflect on your relationship with fat-focused, fat-free and reduced-fat foods. Write in a journal or use the space provided to reflect on the following questions:

What do you believe about food and fat?

_____

_____

_____

_____

How many fat-free or reduced-fat products are in your refrigerator and pantry?

_____

_____

_____

_____

How often do you check fat grams or think about fat content in the food you eat?

_____

_____

_____

_____

How would it feel to stop thinking about fat content?

_____

_____

_____

_____

How do you think that shift would positively impact your Best Energetic Self?

_____

_____

_____

_____

Understanding your relationship with fat-free foods is an essential step in making more conscious choices about incorporating healthy fats into your meals. Healthy fats can make you feel more satiated and improve your focus. You can *trust your process* instead of fad diet rules. In the next section, we'll learn more about the role of healthy fats and the changes I made to support my health.

Healthy Fats Deep Dive

The low-fat craze began as a 1950s hypothesis and, to this day, remains just that—a hypothesis. When people were told to lower their fat intake to reduce the risk of heart attacks, weight gain, and high cholesterol, big food companies started to jump on the trend. They reformulated their products into low-fat versions, feeding the next fad diet wave. With all the mass marketing and packaging, it insidiously became an unquestioned norm.

At the same time, these companies discovered that removing butter and other naturally occurring oils from foods made them more shelf-stable. To compensate for the lost moisture and flavor, hydrogenated oils were manufactured and incorporated to mimic the texture, while sugar and salt were added to enhance flavor. This led to a flood of convenience foods—packaged, mass-produced, and labeled as "diet" options—that still line our grocery store shelves today. The introduction of trans-fats (in the form of partially hydrogenated oils), compounded by the increase in sugar content during this period, has had a devastating effect on heart health. Common products like vegetable shortening, certain popular peanut butter brands, many commercially baked goods and tomato sauces, and coffee creamers contain hydrogenated fats and have become household staples, offering convenience at the expense of our health. Foods with hydrogenated fats that should be limited include soybean oil, seed oils (rapeseed, canola, sunflower), and palm oil, found in many prepared and processed foods.

Seventy percent of our brains are made of fat, so consumption of healthy fats is essential for optimal brain function. Foods with healthy fats that you should eat often include raw and dry-roasted nuts, avocados, olives and olive oil, flax meal, chia seeds, pastured meat and eggs, ghee, coconut oil, and medium-chain triglycerides (MCT).

MCT oil is a type of saturated fat derived from coconut oil that offers several health benefits. MCT oil supports healthy digestion, improves elimination, reduces brain fog, and enhances fat burning. It also helps regulate hunger signals effectively. Unlike other fats,

MCT oil is quickly absorbed into the bloodstream and oxidized by the liver, producing ketones that fuel the brain and body. It's versatile and virtually tasteless, making it an easy addition to smoothies, salad dressings, coffee, tea, and other meals. Note that MCT oil cannot withstand high heat, so it should not be used for cooking. When incorporating MCT oil, start slowly—use one teaspoon at first, and then gradually increase to a tablespoon over the course of a week to allow your body to adjust. Refer to the table below for ideas for including healthy fats in your kitchen.

FANTASTIC FATS	
Choose	Use
Avocados	• Add to salads • Slice one in half and season the avocado as a snack • A bowl with two hard boiled eggs, chopped avocado, tomato, salt and pepper
Cheeses	• Shred over any recipe that inspires you, or use slices with apple or raw veggies for a snack
Whole pasture-raised eggs	• Hard-boiled, fried in ghee, scrambled with a side salad, omelets, or frittata

Whole pasture-raised, beef, pork, chicken	• Roasted, pan-roasted, or shallow-fried...eat the whole piece, including the skin and the fat!
Fatty wild-caught fish	• Lox on sandwiches or eggs, simple salmon or arctic-char dishes, tuna salad (only 12 ounces every week to limit mercury exposure), mackerel tacos
Dry-roasted or raw nuts & seeds	• Add a crunch to salads, tuna salad, chicken salad • Have a handful for a snack • Peanut butter, almond butter, or cashew butter made without hydrogenated fats or added sugar on celery, apple, or carrot • Smoothies • On your steel-cut oats or in chia pudding
Chia seeds	• Chia pudding made with coconut milk or cashew milk

	• Add to salads, smoothies, yogurt, oatmeal
Olive oil	• Use in dressings, marinades, and sauces; not suitable for high heat • Medium-low heat • Roasting is okay
Avocado oil	• Use for cooking with a high smoke point, such as sautéing, frying, or roasting • Avocado mayo
Coconut oil	• Use in high heat, baking, roasting, or stir-fries—Note you will taste the coconut flavor
Ghee	• Use in place of butter as a spread for sautéing vegetables or greasing a pan or skillet
MCT oil	• An easy addition to smoothies, salad dressings, coffee, tea, and other meals. Note that MCT oil cannot withstand high heat, so it should not be used for cooking.

Download this sheet from the book portal to have it on hand!

Quick Look: Trusting Your Process and Healthy Fats

- Write down what "I trust my process" means to you.
- Use the Choose Healthy Fats resource to help you incorporate them into your meals often.
- When you feel a craving for sugar, reach for healthy fats like nuts, seeds, or chia seed pudding (there are plenty of great recipes online).
- Blend MCT oil into salad dressings, tea, or coffee for an extra dose of healthy fat.

Now, let's explore the next affirmation in this chapter.

THINK: *I am the creator of my healthy habits.*

Do you find yourself searching for the perfect program, system, food, or structure to fix your health? The answer you seek is within you. You are the creator of your healthy habits. No meal plan, app, or structure will bring about change for you. The truth is, you are the change. You are the creator. You are the one choosing healthy habits over and over again.

It can feel daunting to realize this truth and to rely solely on yourself and your actions. But ask yourself: What would you do if you weren't afraid to take the next step? What if you already had all the answers? What if those answers helped you build stronger beliefs in yourself instead of carrying the feeling that you aren't living up to some impossible standard?

Sometimes, what I share might feel overwhelming or like the timing isn't right. You may feel hesitant to step into the role of creator, afraid to take even small steps forward. This is especially true when it comes to starting your day. Think about waking up in the morning. Often, our defenses go up as soon as the alarm rings. We tell ourselves we can't get up, that it's too hard. But the truth is, waking up is something you've mastered—you've done it every day of your life. The key isn't just getting out of bed; it's transforming your mornings from something you dread into something you look forward to.

Imagine this: instead of starting the day feeling scattered and unfocused, you wake up with intention, deciding, "I am the creator of my healthy habits." When you embrace this mindset, you step into the day with clarity and focus, ready to take aligned action. The creator within you is present, dialed in, and eager to shape the day ahead. By approaching your mornings this way, you don't just improve your habits—you also sharpen your focus and set the tone for a purposeful and fulfilling day.

To overcome the limitations of your thoughts and personal history with dieting, use the space provided to reflect on what this affirmation means to you.

I am the creator of my healthy habits.

LIVE: *Morning Routines*

My Story

Mornings have never been my strong suit. I'd wake up in a fog, desperately reaching for a triple-shot latte and grabbing whatever quick breakfast I could find at a deli or coffee shop. Caffeine and convenience kept me running, but I wasn't really present—I was just getting through the day. Over time, my routine left me feeling scattered and unmanageable, like I was constantly playing catch-up with my own life. My days blurred together, and no matter how much I pushed through, I couldn't shake the feeling that I was slipping away in the haze. I started to fear that one day, I'd look back and realize I had never truly *been* in my own life—just surviving it. I couldn't live this way anymore. Something had to change.

At first, the changes were small—simply waking up without pressing snooze was a victory. Then, I began walking to work before my coffee, which was about a mile-and-a-half away. Over time, I added more grounding practices, like a journaling exercise and a two-minute meditation. We spend so much time on things that don't serve us, but just a few intentional minutes in the morning can set the tone for the whole day. Waking up and welcoming the day, instead of slogging through it, helps us feel more focused and energized.

For many of us, mornings have become something we dread. We associate them with the stress of waking up, the weight of the news, and the demands of work hanging over our heads. As a result, we look for comfort in the evenings—drinking, watching our favorite shows, and eating late into the night. But what if your mornings, and even your evenings, could become the parts of the day that fill you up instead of drain you? By creating balance in these key times, your body can reset, and your mind may become clear; you can feel more focused throughout the day, making better choices for your health and life.

Morning Routines Inventory

Take a moment to reflect on your relationship with mornings. Write in a journal or use the space provided to reflect on the following questions:

How do you wake up in the morning?

_____

_____

_____

_____

How do you feel first thing in the morning?

_____

_____

_____

_____

What would you like to change about how you feel in the morning?

_____

_____

_____

_____

What is the first thing you would stop doing and the first thing you would start doing to make that change?

_____

_____

_____

_____

How would this positively impact your Best Energetic Self?

_____

_____

_____

_____

Morning Routine Deep Dive

Many people begin their day the same way: rolling out of bed, grabbing their phones, scrolling through social media or email, skipping breakfast, downing coffee, and rushing to work or other responsibilities. Ask yourself: Do you want a more focused life? Do you want to be more productive? Do you want to mindfully reach for your goals? If your answer to all these questions is "yes," the key is to get up powerfully and feel your best earlier. Mornings are a special time when you can fuel the best version of yourself.

I often hear people say, "I'm just not a morning person. I need to sleep." While sleep is essential (and why we need an evening routine), the truth is that you are capable of getting up in the morning and completing a morning routine if you choose to. You can dislike getting up in the morning, yet still do it. An effective morning routine can change your life. It has certainly changed mine from scatter-brained and purposeless to purpose-driven, fulfilling, meaningful, and productive.

To help my clients transform their mornings, I teach a six-step morning practice. This practice follows the acronym, "SISTER" and is designed to align the mind and body with *Energetic Eating*. You can complete this routine in as little as 15 minutes. Sometimes you will have time for only a few of the steps, and that's okay! Choose the ones that make sense for you.

Silence (1 minute). Begin your day quietly. Don't pick up your phone or engage with anyone yet—just sit in stillness. Remove yourself from the bedroom if needed. You might turn on the coffee maker if it's prepared, but avoid jumping into the ritual or drinking it. Simply breathe or listen to a short meditation. Start with one minute if longer feels challenging.

I am (2 minutes). Reflect on your Best Energetic Self from the writing exercise in Chapter 3. (It's even better if you print it out or have it handy in your journal.) What positive words do you need to hear today to embody that version of yourself? What part of your Best Energetic Self do you want to actualize today, this week, or this year? Write your affirmations and intentions using "I am" statements in the present tense, as if they are *already* happening. (I am usually drinking coffee by now!)

Show Me (2 minutes). Picture yourself as your Best Energetic Self—standing tall, smiling confidently, and radiating wellness. Visualize the choices you'll make throughout the day to nourish and support this version of your. Add "show me" statements to invite clarity, guidance, and opportunities from the universe. These statements show you *how, who, what, when,* or *where* the "I am" affirmation will unfold. They transform your affirmation into an active request, letting the universe guide you toward the manifestation in tangible ways.

Take Action (5–30 min). Choose an activity that helps you embody your Best Energetic Self. This could be any kind of movement like stretching, yoga, or a walk—exercise is a good choice if this is the only time of day you can get it in. Or choose creative expression through reading, listening to a podcast, or simply setting up your space for the day ahead. The goal is to align your actions with the energy and mindset you've cultivated. Whether you spend two minutes or 30, let this be a conscious practice that connects you with your vision and sets a positive tone for everything that follows.

Express Gratitude (2 minutes). Write down what you feel grateful for— anything that brings you joy or appreciation. Practicing gratitude is a simple yet powerful way to elevate your mood, shift your energy in a positive direction, and ground you in a mindset of possibility before you take your next step.

Reread (3 minutes). Take a moment to review what you just wrote, along with previous morning journal entries. Look for any signs that what you've asked for is unfolding and write them down. This step reinforces your trust and belief in the process, shifting your mindset from doubt to expectation to recognition. Noticing even small progress helps you recognize synchronicities, mindset shifts, and tangible results. This reflection builds momentum, reinforcing that your intentions are taking shape and keeping you motivated and aligned with your goals.

You can access a printable sheet for this routine in the portal.

Tips for success in implementing your morning routine:

- Wake up 15 minutes earlier than usual, and don't press snooze.
- Choose a space that feels good for your morning routine.
- Plan your evening routine to ensure you get enough sleep to make the morning routine happen.

Quick Look: Creating Healthy Habits and Morning Routines

- Reflect on what it means to be the creator of your healthy habits.
- Download and print the SISTER routine from the portal to have on hand.

Disclaimer: If you feel you are experiencing severe and unresolved brain fog or attention issues that are negatively impacting your life, seek professional help from a doctor or health practitioner.

The Power of Conscious Choices with Your Focus

I went from believing that a low-fat diet was the key to weight loss to consciously choosing healthy fats that support my brain. Now, I add MCT oil to my coffee, enrich my meals with olive oil and avocado, snack on nuts and seeds, and cook with ghee and avocado oil. I went from barely holding my life together to joyfully waking up in the morning, ready to take on my goals. Mornings have become my favorite time to be with myself, exercise, and prepare for a productive day. Waking up before my alarm feels natural, and I start my day with purpose instead of focusing on the scale.

That sense of clarity and ease wasn't always my reality—and I've seen the same struggle in my clients. One client, in particular, came to me for help with weight loss, but it quickly became clear that the issue wasn't just about food or exercise—it was about feeling completely out of control in her daily life. She was stuck in an unbalanced cycle, trying to manage everything but herself.

At first glance, she seemed to be doing all the right things—working out twice a week and making what she believed were healthy food choices. But as we peeled back the layers, a different story emerged. Each morning, she dragged herself out of bed, weighed herself, and reached straight for coffee, running on autopilot as she got her kids ready for school. She'd rush through her workout, squeeze in a quick shower, and dive into meetings—sometimes even with wet hair.

Her attention was locked on losing weight, but what we uncovered was far more significant: she needed to stop the anxiety-driven hustle and reclaim her mornings. Together, we worked on incorporating components of the SISTER practice. She started eating breakfast, adding healthy fats like avocado, nuts, and eggs to fuel her brain and stabilize her energy throughout the day. Her morning energy went from chaos to calm.

The results were transformative. She became more focused, clear-headed, and moved through her day with greater ease. Her relationship with herself changed—she began speaking to herself with compassion instead of criticism. And as her mindset shifted, so did her body. Her energy improved, her stress diminished, and her body began working *for* her instead of *against* her.

This journey wasn't about adding more tasks—it was about creating space for what truly mattered. It was about shifting focus from just losing weight to nurturing her well-being, allowing her body and mind to find balance again.

That's the power of reclaiming your focus—when you align your choices with your Best Energetic Self, your whole life begins to flow with more ease, clarity, and joy.

When you first start incorporating these affirmations, habits, routines, and rituals, you may feel some resistance. Most people don't want to give up their current habits, even when those habits leave them feeling scattered, foggy, or unmotivated. In the *Energetic Eating Method*, I help clients recognize how their food and lifestyle choices impact their focus and sense of control over their day.

Remember to ask yourself: What would my Best Energetic Self want me to do?

This is the foundation of making conscious choices for your focus. It's about creating calm and awareness first thing in the morning, and choosing to add healthy fats to your meals. Here's what that looks like:

- Recognizing how food impacts mental clarity before making a choice. Instead of grabbing something just because it's convenient or familiar, pause. Ask yourself: How does this meal support my ability to focus? Will this fuel

sustained energy or leave me drained? Choosing healthy fats—like avocado, nuts, seeds, and omega-rich foods—can be an act of self-care, a way to nourish the brain and keep you sharp throughout the day.
- Understanding that there's a time for structure and a time for flexibility. Some mornings thrive on routine—waking up early, hydrating, moving your body, and fueling with a nourishing meal. Other days, your Best Energetic Self may need more rest or a slower start. Rather than forcing yourself into a rigid schedule, make morning choices that support you, not control you.
- Allowing mornings to be intentional, not stressful. Instead of waking up feeling behind or reacting to external pressures, shift into a proactive mindset. Mornings are an opportunity to center yourself, set the tone for the day, and take a moment to check in with your body. A rushed, chaotic morning does not define the rest of your day—conscious choices can shift everything.

I know it's okay to skip my morning routine when my body needs extra rest, without guilt or feeling like I've failed. I also know it's okay to indulge in an easy, comforting breakfast sometimes, as long as I do it with awareness. Missing one structured morning doesn't mean I've lost my progress—it means I'm staying connected to what I truly need. This is the real shift—from rules to self-trust, from restriction to alignment, from reacting to choosing. Every day is a new opportunity to listen, honor, and decide what serves you best.

Use the *Energetic Eating* journaling exercise to explore how making conscious choices from this chapter can help you. Prompts are provided in the journal to guide you if you feel stuck.

Date: _____

MIT(s): *What is the most important thing you'd like to focus on from your Best Energetic Self?*		
How I Think:	How I Eat:	How I Live:
What is a positive thought or affirmation that you would like to take with you?	*When you think about supporting yourself nutritionally, what could that look like now?*	*When you think about supporting yourself through lifestyle choices, what could that look like now?*

Breakfast: How did you feel?	
Lunch: How did you feel?	
Dinner: How did you feel?	
Snack 1: How did you feel?	Snack 2: How did you feel?
Liquids: How did you feel?	
Reflection on Conscious Choices: *How are you feeling today? What conscious choices did you make with your thoughts, eating, and lifestyle?*	

CHAPTER 8
PILLAR 5: YOUR ENERGY LEVELS

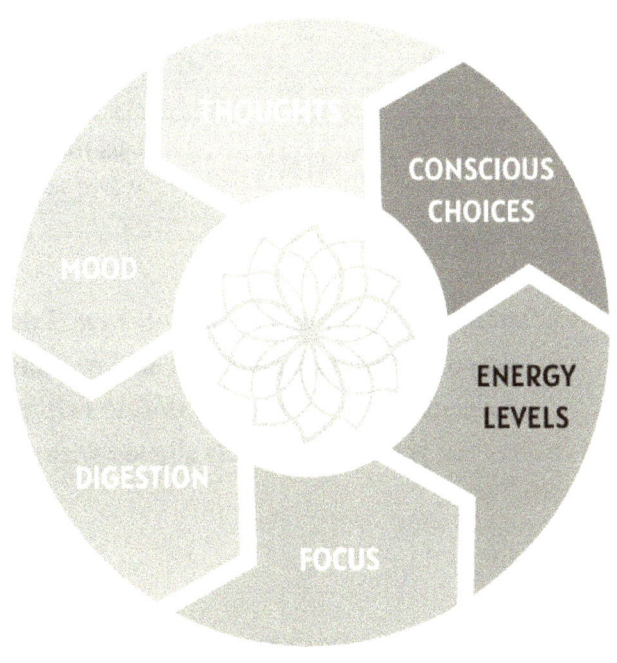

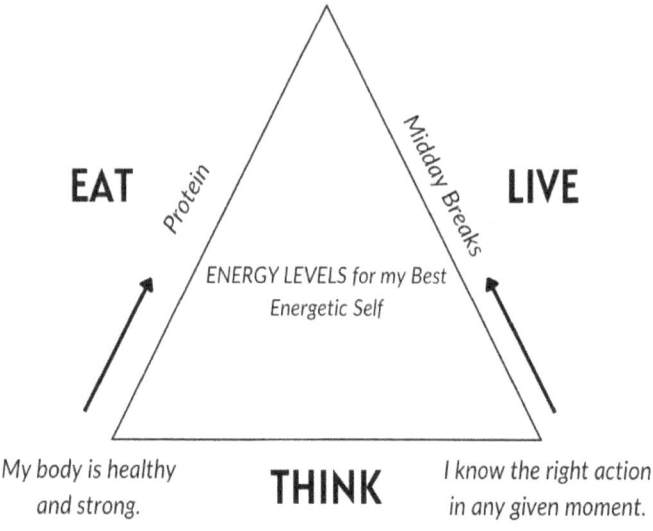

In this chapter, through the Think, Eat, Live Triad, we'll explore two empowering affirmations, a key nutritional component, and a transformative lifestyle shift to help you make conscious choices for your energy levels aligned with your Best Energetic Self.

Overview

Energy drain has many root causes, but we often misplace the blame. We might attribute it to laziness, an overwhelming schedule, or the demands of daily life. Sometimes, we believe it's because of our heavier bodies and think weight loss is the solution when, in reality, we simply don't have the energy to take action in the first place. The truth is energy loss doesn't happen overnight—it's a gradual process that builds over time. For many women, it's the result of cumulative choices and stressors that eventually push the body to its breaking point. Cortisol levels spike, stress responses go into overdrive, sleep becomes disrupted, blood sugar crashes, and eating patterns spiral out of control, leaving us stuck in a cycle of exhaustion.

In this pillar, we'll explore how protein balances our energy and prevents our reliance on quick fixes like sugar and refined carbohydrates that actually deplete our energy levels. We will also see that stress and overwork play major roles in energy depletion. Being in "work mode" 24/7 raises cortisol levels, disrupting multiple systems in your body. High cortisol signals the need for more insulin, which disrupts glucose regulation and leads to more cravings. This cycle slows our metabolism and can eventually cause insulin resistance. Adequate protein, amino-acid intake, and stress management can signal your body to regulate hunger, support metabolic function, and restore energy. To support this process, we'll explore two empowering affirmations (Think), the importance of protein (Eat), and midday breaks to reset and recharge (Live).

Energy Levels Reflection

Rate each of the following on a scale of 1–5, with 1 meaning "never," 3 meaning "sometimes," and 5 meaning "always." Consider these questions in relation to the past six months.

- *Do you experience energy dips during the day?*
- *Do you wake up feeling tired?*
- *Do you often skip meals?*
- *Do you rely on sugar or processed food for energy?*
- *Do you struggle to settle into sleep at night?*

Total: ___ out of 25

If you scored 15 or higher, the suggestions in this chapter will be especially helpful for you to explore and implement.

Now, let's explore the affirmations, nutrition, and lifestyle strategies that will support your energy levels.

THINK: *My body is healthy and strong.*

Being healthy and strong is a mindset, not just an end goal. Too often, we are conditioned to seek external markers—like a specific number, size, or image—that we believe define health and strength. These ideas of optimal health are arbitrary, rooted in comparison rather than connection to your core self.

You might compare yourself to an old photo, someone you follow on social media, a friend or a family member, or even an advertisement. But these comparisons only distract from what your body can do today. Instead of focusing on what you can't do, or who you are not, I encourage you to take joyful action based on what you can do and who you are. One of the most powerful ways to support this mindset is through nourishment, and protein plays a key role.

Protein is the nutrient of strength. It isn't just about muscle—it's about resilience, recovery, and vitality. Every cell in your body relies on protein to repair, regenerate, and function optimally. When you prioritize high-quality protein sources, you're actively supporting your body's strength and health from the inside out. You're sending a message to yourself that you are worth nourishing, that your body is capable, and that strength is something you cultivate daily—not something you wait to achieve.

On the other hand, if you tell yourself your body is not healthy or strong, you will meet yourself with that energy and have a hard time taking positive steps forward. But when you shift into the belief that your body is already strong, your choices naturally follow—whether it's fueling yourself with protein to support muscle recovery, stabilizing energy levels, or simply giving your body what it needs to thrive. This is how true strength is built: not just in the body, but in the mind.

To overcome the limitations of your thoughts and personal history with dieting, use the space provided to reflect on what this affirmation means to you.

My body is healthy and strong.

Now that you've explored what it means to be healthy and strong, let's explore the "Eat" portion of the triad as it relates to energy levels.

EAT: *Prioritize Protein*

My Story

Seven years before I gave up fad dieting, I was juggling a full-time job as a school teacher, attending graduate school, and parenting a two-year-old. I was so. Freaking. Tired.

Every day, around 2:00 p.m., my energy levels would plummet. My life felt completely unmanageable. Domestic chores piled on top of work for the next day. I would come home around 5:00 p.m. and collapse face-first into bed for a few minutes of quiet before starting Mom duty. I blamed it all on my work demands, thinking I had no control over my schedule whatsoever.

At the same time, I was also following a 90-day total body program. My mornings started with shakes and my meals were meticulously portioned into containers for carbs, fats, and proteins. It wasn't that the food itself was bad—but the rigid portioning created obsessive and unsustainable habits. I was so strict about portions that I couldn't tune in to my hunger or fullness cues. Whatever fit into the container was all I could eat, even if my body needed more. I was in a constant state of deprivation, trying to control my body for the sake of weight loss instead of listening to what it actually needed.

Looking back, I wish I'd known then what I know now. Protein is essential in the long game of sustaining energy levels and repairing the body on a foundational level. Instead of limiting my food intake to containers and shakes, I could have focused on getting enough protein to fuel my busy life.

After a few weeks, I gave up on the 90-day program. It was too complicated to maintain on top of my already hectic schedule, and I was tired and hungry all the time. I realized I didn't have to live in a constant state of hunger, deprivation, or lethargy. Consuming more protein didn't negatively impact my health or weight-loss goals—in fact, it supported them. Choosing diets that limited how much I ate no longer made sense because I could focus on eating with a mindset of abundance rather than scarcity. Thanks to adequate protein intake in a balanced meal, my body is now healthy and strong and my energy levels are sustained, making it possible to repair muscles and refuel after workouts.

Protein Inventory

Let's take inventory of your relationship with eating protein. Write in a journal or use the space provided to reflect on the following questions:

Do you turn to diets that hyper-focus on calorie intake, such as portioning or calorie counting?

_____
_____
_____
_____

How does inadequate protein intake impact your energy levels and feelings of satiety?

_____
_____
_____
_____

What would you like to change about your consumption of protein?

_____
_____
_____
_____

What do you think would be the first step in making that change?

_____

_____

_____

How would restoring your energy levels positively impact your Best Energetic Self?

_____

_____

_____

Protein Deep Dive

Protein plays a vital role in our bodies by reducing hunger hormones and increasing satiety. While some diets overemphasize protein intake—leading to digestive distress, weight gain, and elimination of healthy carbohydrates—most women I work with struggle to get enough protein, which often shows up as energy crashes during the day.

Both vegetable and animal proteins support the body, but it's important to note the differences. Many vegetarian protein sources lack a complete essential amino acid profile, which is needed for breaking down food, building and repairing muscle mass (key for metabolism), repairing tissue, and producing usable energy. For vegetarians, it's essential to get protein intake from sources like beans, lentils, legumes, chia seeds, edamame, and healthy carbohydrates such as quinoa, bulgur, and farro. If you're following an unprocessed vegetarian diet and still feel tired, consider working with a coach, nutritionist, or dietitian to explore adjustment.

When I was vegetarian, the foods and lifestyle didn't work for my body, and I was the unhealthiest I'd ever been. Like me, you might benefit from incorporating sustainably sourced, free-range chicken, grass-fed beef, or wild-caught fish into your diet. It's important to note that I ultimately *had* to leave strict vegetarianism behind for my Best Energetic Self, so my perspective in this chapter is influenced by that experience. Keep in mind, however, that everyone's body is different. No matter what you choose, I believe it's important that it aligns with your body and Best Energetic Self.

When planning meals, think about protein as about one quarter of a balanced plate. Here are some examples to help you think about what this could look like:

- 1 pasture-raised chicken thigh, ¼ plate roasted sweet potatoes, ½ plate salad
- ½ plate rice and beans, ½ plate vegetables.
- A stir-fry with ½ plate broccoli, mushrooms, snow peas, and onions; ¼ plate quinoa; ¼ plate lentils or grass-fed beef.
- ¼ plate palm-sized pork chop or loin, ¼ plate roasted potatoes, ½ plate Brussels sprouts.
- ¼ plate hummus, ¼ plate warm bulgur, and ½ plate vegetables.
- Low-mercury wild-caught fish paired with ½ plate sautéed vegetables, ¼ plate quinoa, and ¼ plate of salad.

Not all proteins are created equal. Focus on high-quality animal proteins and organic, unprocessed vegetarian proteins. Avoid highly processed options, particularly processed soy-based products, which can play an outsized role in vegetarian diets.

As we have discussed, your Best Energetic Self is the culmination of your thoughts, your food, and your lifestyle. Choosing proteins cultivated with care, such as local, organic, grass-fed, pastured meat and eggs, support your body and well-being. The real issue isn't plant-based versus animal-based diets; it's the industrialization and commercialization of highly processed, genetically modified foods that often contain indigestible ingredients. Listening to your body, prioritizing a varied diet, and choosing minimally processed, nutrient-dense foods can make a profound difference in how you feel.

To help you make healthy protein choices, I've included a table below and in the book portal. Use it to identify cleaner protein options that maximize nutrient intake, essential amino acids, and digestibility for sustained energy.

PRIORITIZING PROTEINS	
Choose	Lose
Grass-fed and pasture-raised beef, pork, chicken	The USDA uses words like prime, choice, select, and standard; these only refer to the amount of usable meat, not the treatment of the animal

Pastured eggs (a.k.a Pasture-Raised)	On its own, organic can mean anything. Organic feed, for example, could be by-products. It also doesn't indicate a free-roaming life
Low-mercury and sustainably-harvested fish: wild-caught salmon, mackerel, anchovies, sardines, herring, clams, mussels, oysters, gulf shrimp	Fish to be mindful of due to high mercury or sustainability concerns: Swordfish, shark, grouper, Chilean sea bass, halibut, tuna
Protein powders with minimal ingredients and no added sugars, such as pea protein paired with rice protein, whey protein, egg white protein	Soy protein

Quick Look: Health, Strength, and Protein for Energy Levels

- Reflect on what it means to you to be healthy and strong.
- Include proteins with your meals and snacks to help regulate your energy levels throughout the day.
- Refer to the list of protein sources and visit the book portal for a printable version.

Now, let's move on to the second affirmation of this chapter: *I know the right action at any given moment.*

THINK: *I know the right action at any given moment.*

How often have you felt stuck, unsure if the choice you're about to make will harm or help you? What would it be like to trust that the choices you make are in your best interest, no matter what?

The issue isn't the choice itself—it's the time we spend worrying about whether something is "good" or "bad," whether we're eating too many calories, avoiding enough fat, or exercising enough. Knowing the right action means making thoughtful—not obsessive—choices. And even if you make a "wrong" choice, it's okay. Every choice is a chance to learn. Instead of feeling guilty, you can simply say, "*Now I know more.*"

However, if you repeatedly make choices that don't serve you, it's time for reflection. Making the right choice is about seizing opportunities to learn—not acting out of fear of change or giving in to self-sabotage. Be honest and clear with yourself about your motivations.

Fad diets perpetuate the idea that we can't trust ourselves to make choices on our own and that health and weight loss are all about the "right" foods and maintaining a macronutrient deficit. This creates unnecessary anxiety over our decisions. Instead, let's shift the narrative: *you can tune in to the right action at any given moment and honor your Best Energetic Self.*

And one of the simplest ways to do this is by taking midday breaks.

When you pause—whether it's stepping away from your work, eating a balanced meal, stretching, or even closing your eyes for a few minutes—you're reinforcing the belief that you can trust yourself. Instead of pushing through exhaustion or ignoring your body's cues, you're making a thoughtful choice that supports your energy and well-being.

A midday break isn't just about resting—it's about realigning with yourself. It's a moment to check in and ask: *What do I need right now?* Maybe it's a protein-rich snack to keep your energy steady, a walk to reset your mind, or simply a few deep breaths to shift your energy. These small choices, made with intention, build trust in yourself and your ability to care for your body.

To overcome the limitations of your thoughts and personal history with dieting, use the space provided to reflect on what this affirmation means to you.

I know the right action at any given moment.

Now that you've explored what it means to know the right action at any given moment, let's move to the "Live" portion of the triad and dive into the importance of midday breaks.

LIVE: *Include Midday Breaks*

My Story

Taking a break used to mean stepping outside the office for a cigarette. When I worked as an Associate Producer for a TV show in New York in my 20s, smoking was one of the only socially acceptable excuses to step away. Looking back, I can see how treating breaks as weaknesses leads us to develop habits that feel like they *need* to happen, such as smoking, grabbing coffee, checking social media, or reaching for a snack. These habits might seem replenishing at the moment, but they often drain more energy than they restore. Even though I don't smoke anymore, I still love a good cup of coffee. But I've learned that when I reach for a second or third cup instead of taking a restorative break, I feel worse by the end of the day.

The challenge is to find ways to take breaks that actually replenish you—whether that's through breathing exercises, closing your eyes, or moving your body. You can use these pauses to reset and ask yourself: *What is the right action for me in this moment?*

Midday Breaks Inventory

Take a moment to reflect on your relationship with breaks. Write in a journal or use the space provided to reflect on the following questions:

How do you feel in the middle of the day?

_____

_____

_____

_____

What would you like to change about how you feel during that time?

_____

_____

_____

_____

What is one thing you could stop doing that depletes energy?

_____

_____

_____

_____

What is one thing you could start doing to gain energy?

_____

_____

_____

_____

How would these changes positively impact your Best Energetic Self?

_____

_____

_____

_____

Midday Breaks Deep Dive

Many of us associate taking breaks with laziness, but taking breaks—like a good sleep routine—is essential for productivity and well-being. One of the most limiting beliefs we hold is that "breaks take too much time." In reality, rest and productivity are two sides of the same coin. So, number one, drop the idea that breaks are unproductive and instead, embrace them as *necessary*. Taking intentional, high-quality breaks is what sets you apart as a high performer rather than someone stuck in a cycle of burnout.

Chronic stress and perpetual work elevate cortisol levels, which can wreak havoc on thyroid and reproductive hormones, blood pressure, the immune system, memory, and metabolism. High cortisol levels send signals to your body that it needs to slow down to cope with the stress—slowing your metabolism, increasing your cravings, and leaving you feeling fatigued.

When we think about work and rest, we tend to picture a wave of ups and downs. But I want you to imagine rest differently—not as a "down" moment, but as something just as productive as work itself. Instead of a wave, imagine a steady line of intentional effort—both at work and at rest. This is not the kind of rest where you collapse onto the couch thinking, "Oh gosh, I have to lie down because I hate my life." That's the point we want to avoid. Your body thrives when you're a productive rester, not someone on a slow decline to burnout.

You actually do your best work when your brain is trained to shift into recovery mode rather than burnout mode. However, you have to be mindful of "rest" activities that may actually rev you up and drain your energy—like scrolling on your phone, mindless snacking, or aimless distractions. You can maximize productivity in a way that aligns with your goals, whether that's work, exercise, parenting, or other conscious choices that support your Best Energetic Self.

Intentional solitude and digital breaks give your brain the space it needs to roam freely—to find creativity, peace, and meaning. The recommended balance is to work 50–90 minutes and then take a recovery break lasting 10–20 minutes. When I was writing this book, I would set a timer for 50 minutes and then take a break by walking outside, grabbing a glass of water, or practicing a progressive relaxation. You'll need to experiment to find what works for you; some days, I choose to focus for only 20 minutes before I take a pause.

Now, think for a moment: How much time do you spend on energy-sucking breaks? Maybe you pick up a snack you don't really need, feel guilty about it, and lose five minutes. Maybe you scroll on your phone and suddenly realize you've forgotten something important after 20 minutes. We all have pockets of time throughout the day that slip away from us. The trick is to notice when it happens and replace those moments with more high-performing breaks that actually replenish you.

Imagine if you worked as hard on breaks as you do at your job. What would change if your body could shift out of stress mode and into true recovery? Explore the examples below to see how impactful intentional breaks can be.

Midday Breaks to Decrease Stress and Sustain Energy

- Listen to a song: Choose one that matches your mood. Need a happiness boost? Or calm reflection? Play it, but don't touch your phone during the music.
- Stand up and stretch then sit back down, relax your shoulders and jaw, close your eyes or look out a window, and take a few deep breaths.
- Go for a quick walk. Even five minutes can have an impact on your energy levels.
- Create a coffee or tea ritual: If it's before 1 p.m., enjoy a mindful moment preparing matcha, a cappuccino, or your favorite green tea. Later in the day, you can try other kinds of enlivening herbal teas, such as peppermint or orange.
- Journal. Open a journal and free-write. If you're stuck, start with an affirmation like "I am healthy. I am powerful. I am connected," or jot down five things you're grateful for.
- Try a quick meditation.
- Body scan: Set a timer for 10–20 minutes. Mentally relax each part of your body, starting from your toes and working up to the crown of your head, ending with deep, grounding breaths.
- Rub your hands together and create heat then gently place your hands over your eyes, creating dark pockets for your eyes to rest in the center of your palms. Take a few deep breaths.

Visit the portal to download and print out the Midday Breaks Resource to keep at your desk or in a favorite resting spot at home. I have also included a video demonstrating a tapping point to increase energy and focus.

Quick Look: Taking Right Action and Midday Breaks

- Reflect on what it means to take the right action at any given moment.
- Choose three ways you can replace low-performing breaks with high-performing breaks.
- Try the tapping point for increased energy in the portal.

Disclaimer: If you feel you are experiencing uneven energy throughout the day or low energy levels that can't be resolved with food and lifestyle, seek professional help from a doctor or health practitioner.

The Power of Conscious Choices for Your Energy Levels

Today, I move through my day feeling energized and steady, without the need to lie down or take a nap. By prioritizing protein and integrating brief, intentional midday breaks, I've been able to avoid those once-familiar energy dips. On the rare occasion my body feels worn out, I now know how to recharge effectively using the midday breaks from this chapter.

This balance has transformed my ability to be present and engaged with my kids when they come home from school. Whether it's playing with them or helping with homework, I can say yes to more throughout the day because I'm no longer weighed down by constant fatigue. Feeling less overwhelmed has allowed me to embrace life with more energy and presence.

I've seen this same shift happen for my clients, many of whom come to me struggling with dragging energy and stubborn weight fluctuations. The *2 p.m. slump* is a common complaint—one that often stretches into the evening and leaves them feeling too depleted to enjoy life or even prepare a nourishing meal.

This was the case for one of my clients, a dedicated executive managing a high-pressure career. Her days were packed with back-to-back meetings, leaving little time for herself. Lunch was often a rushed sandwich in between calls. By the time she got home, she'd throw together an easy pasta dinner for her kids with her partner and collapse into bed—only to wake up the next morning and do it all over again.

Her exhaustion was more than just physical—it was a clear indicator that something needed to change. At first, she believed that working harder made her more valuable, that pushing through her fatigue was a sign of dedication. But as we worked together, it became clear that her mindset—and her energy management—were keeping her stuck.

We started with one simple shift: creating space for midday breaks. Instead of powering through the afternoon, she began stepping away from her desk to enjoy meals she prepared the night before—meals centered around the palm-sized portion of protein her body was desperately asking for, rather than the refined carbs from her daily sandwiches.

She began walking after lunch, giving her body the chance to balance her blood sugar and soak up much-needed vitamin D. These seemingly small changes created powerful results. Her energy stabilized, her productivity soared, and she found herself carrying that renewed energy into her evenings—spending quality time with her kids and feeling present instead of depleted.

But the biggest transformation wasn't just physical—it was in how she saw herself. She realized that years of cycling through fad diets and ignoring her body's needs had kept her stuck in a loop of frustration. Once she began addressing her energy levels instead of just focusing on the scale, everything changed. She felt lighter, freer, and more capable of sustaining the life she wanted to live.

That's the real key to unlocking your energy—shifting from survival mode to intentional living. When you prioritize your body's needs and honor your natural rhythms, you'll discover a level of energy that empowers you to show up fully for yourself and those you love.

When you first start incorporating these affirmations, habits, routines, and rituals, you may feel some resistance. Most people don't want to give up their current patterns, even when they leave them feeling drained. In the *Energetic Eating Method*, clients prioritize their energy, so healthier choices come easily. Many share that having more energy not only makes them feel better but also creates more time to enjoy the people and activities they love. It's not just about protein or midday breaks—it's about reclaiming the energy to fully embrace life.

Remember to ask yourself: What would my Best Energetic Self want me to do?

This is the foundation of making conscious choices for your energy levels. It's about prioritizing protein and choosing rest from a place of empowerment rather than the fear of falling behind. Here's what that looks like:

- Recognizing when your body needs nourishment versus rest. Instead of pushing through fatigue with caffeine or sugar, pause. Ask yourself: Do I need protein for sustained energy, or would a short break help me reset? Understanding the difference allows you to make choices that fuel you instead of depleting you.
- Understanding that there's a time to prioritize protein and a time to listen to other cues. Some days, your body will benefit from a protein-rich meal to maintain energy and satiety. Other times, the most supportive choice might be slowing down, stretching, or stepping outside for fresh air. Learning to balance both is key to feeling truly energized.
- Allowing breaks to be restorative, not guilt-inducing. Midday breaks are not a sign of weakness or laziness—they are tools for sustainable energy. Instead of viewing rest as a disruption, see it as an essential part of productivity and well-being. A ten-minute reset can shift your entire afternoon.

I know it's a form of nourishment to take a break when my body signals that it needs one, without guilt or the pressure to do more. I also know it's okay to have a day where my energy isn't perfect—because I trust myself to nourish and recharge in a way that supports me.

Use the *Energetic Eating* journaling exercise below to reflect on how the conscious choices from this chapter can support your Best Energetic Self. Prompts are included in the journal to guide you if you feel stuck.

This is the real shift—from rules to self-trust, from restriction to alignment, from reacting to choosing. Every day is a new opportunity to listen, honor, and decide what serves you best.

Date: _____

MIT(s): *What is the most important thing you'd like to focus on from your Best Energetic Self?*		
How I Think:	How I Eat:	How I Live:
What is a positive thought or affirmation that you would like to take with you?	*When you think about supporting yourself nutritionally, what could that look like now?*	*When you think about supporting yourself through lifestyle choices, what could that look like now?*

Breakfast:
How did you feel?
Lunch:
How did you feel?
Dinner:
How did you feel?

Snack 1:	Snack 2:
How did you feel?	How did you feel?

Liquids:
How did you feel?
Reflection on Conscious Choices: *How are you feeling today? What conscious choices did you make with your thoughts, eating, and lifestyle?*

CHAPTER 9

PILLAR 6: CONSCIOUS CHOICES

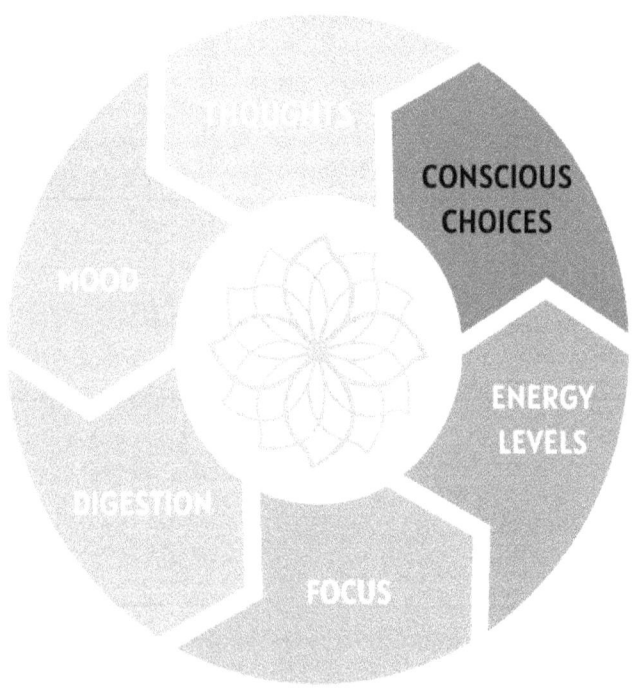

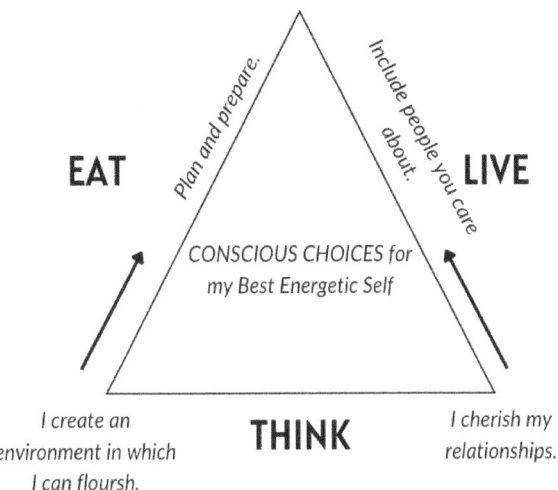

In this chapter, through the Think, Eat, Live Triad, we'll explore two empowering affirmations, a key nutritional component, and a transformative lifestyle shift to help you deepen conscious choices aligned with your Best Energetic Self.

Overview

Welcome to the final pillar: Conscious Choices. Throughout the pillars, you've learned how to make conscious choices to support your Best Energetic Self and strengthen your Triad of Health using the five pillars: Thoughts, Mood, Digestion, Focus, and Energy Levels. This final pillar, Conscious Choices, is the key to maintaining the strength of the triad. By tuning into your body and intentionally choosing to strengthen these pillars through your thoughts, foods, and lifestyle, you can continue to nurture your Best Energetic Self. Additionally, setting yourself up for success in your environment and within your relationships will help you sustain these choices over time.

The most important aspect of conscious choices is identifying how you are making them. Indulgences can absolutely be a part of your life—as long as you pay close attention to how they affect the pillars of health. For example, I enjoy watching TV, but if I binge for hours, I can't perform my best the next day, nor do I have the energy to exercise. Recognizing that gives me the *why* for my conscious choice to turn the TV off: I'm preserving my energy for tomorrow.

Understanding your *why* is equally important when you choose to indulge. For instance, I can enjoy a cupcake if I approach it with a mindset of savoring the experience. If I eat it from a place of guilt, however, I know that guilt will likely spiral into skipping exercise or making "screw it" choices for the rest of the day. Next time you make a conscious choice, take a moment to examine *why*.

Conscious choices align with who you are (your Best Energetic Self) and how you want to feel—avoiding the discomforts of disrupted thoughts, mood, digestion, focus, or energy levels. Think of it as data collection rather than judgment. There's no need to get your emotions involved. You're learning what supports your Best Energetic Self.

Sometimes, the best choice for you is one that the rest of the world might label "unhealthy." The rules aren't theirs to make; they're yours. The guidance you need comes from within you.

Use the flowchart below to help you gain more clarity each time you make a conscious choice using what you've learned about supporting the triad with the other pillars of health.

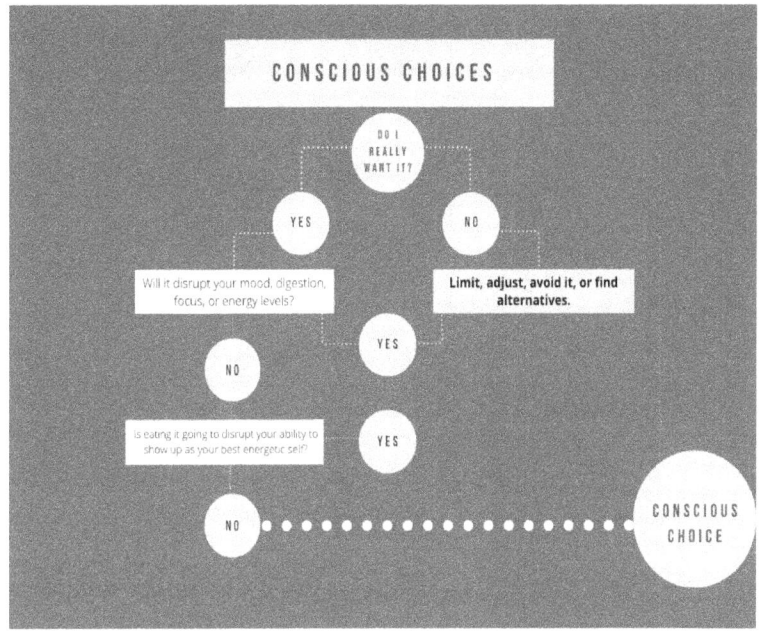

In the beginning, you may find yourself putting a lot of thought into making conscious choices, talking yourself through the process step by step, almost like mapping it out in your mind. But over time, it will become second nature. What initially takes 30 seconds of consideration will eventually become effortless, taking just a moment, until it becomes an integral part of who you are.

Conscious Choices Reflection

Rate each of the following on a scale of 1–5, with 1 meaning "never," 3 meaning "sometimes," and 5 meaning "always." Consider these questions in relation to the past six months.

- Do you ignore your body's mood, digestion, focus, and energy level signals?
- Do you forget to consider how your choices affect your ability to show up as your Best Self?

- Do time, circumstances, work, friends, or family life often distract you from making conscious choices for your health and well-being?
- Do you avoid conscious food choices such as making or preparing food because you feel unsupported or overwhelmed?
- Do you find yourself avoiding healthy lifestyle choices like sleep and exercise for similar reasons?

Total: ___ out of 25

If you scored 15 or higher, the suggestions in this chapter will be especially helpful for you to explore and implement.

Now, let's explore the affirmations, nutrition, and lifestyle strategies that will support you in making conscious choices.

THINK: *I create an environment in which I can flourish.*

Too often, we give our power away to situational or environmental stress. Constraints like not having the right food, time, equipment, or setting often stop us from taking action for our Best Energetic Selves. However, allowing the environment to control you, rather than creating an environment where you can flourish, is a decision made out of fear or perfectionism. Things don't need to be "just so" for you to thrive.

Creating supportive environments for your health and well-being is simpler than it seems. Examples include surrounding yourself with helpful tools and resources, like buying groceries that align with your goals, placing your yoga mat next to the bed or in front of the TV, setting your workout clothes out the night before, or prepping your lunch for the next day. These small habits enable you to make conscious choices when the time comes.

But what happens when your environment is less than ideal? What do you do when things feel out of control? Maybe your partner comes home late, your family serves a meal that doesn't work for you, it's 8 p.m. and you haven't exercised, or you overslept that morning. These moments happen to everyone, but the difference lies in your response. Tell yourself that you can flourish within the constraints of your situation.

For example, during a home renovation, our family didn't have a kitchen for three months—just a tiny table, microwave, an instant pot, and a blender. We could have used this as an excuse to eat out every day or rely on convenience foods. Instead, we chose to rise to the challenge. We made smoothies in the morning, salads in the afternoon, and instant pot meals in the evening. When we ordered out, we selected foods that helped us thrive and stretched those meals by using the leftovers.

Diet mentality teaches us that life circumstances can derail our conscious choices, sending us into the all-or-nothing and black-and-white mentality. When things don't go perfectly, we abandon our intentions. To overcome this mindset, believe in your ability to create an environment where you can flourish. Flourishing doesn't always have to be 100%. At times of challenge, flourishing might be 74%. Or even 40%. But that's miles better than throwing in the towel and doing nothing. You can find ways to make the most of the real situations you face.

Use the provided space to reflect on what this affirmation means to you.

I create an environment in which I can flourish.

Now that you've explored what it means to create an environment in which you can flourish, let's dive into the "Eat" portion of the triad and how it connects to conscious choices.

EAT: *Plan and Prepare Based on the Pillars*

My Story

Do you ever feel like you're making every excuse to avoid taking better care of yourself? Maybe you sleep in, order takeout, or stay up late, and you're left wondering whether you're truly honoring your health or just making excuses?

This is how I lived for years, constantly searching for diets to undo the damage from choices that didn't serve me. I didn't know how to listen to my body's cues or take the right steps toward self-care. When I felt sad or depressed, I'd turn to sugar. When I had digestive discomfort, I'd throw in the towel and eat poorly anyway. When I felt unfocused or scattered, I'd excuse myself from work and grab a convenience food. And when my energy was low, I sought a quick fix through coffee or sweets.

I wasn't making conscious choices to support my well-being in the long run—I was chasing temporary relief. I blamed everything—time, money, energy—but the truth was, I had the power to take charge of my health. I just needed to create a physical space inside of my body and in my surroundings that set me up for success. I will give more examples later in this chapter.

Your Conscious Choices Eating Inventory

Let's take inventory of your conscious choices. Write in a journal or use the space provided to reflect on the following questions:

When do you ignore your body's signals, such as fullness, hunger, moodiness, digestive issues, lack of focus, or energy levels?

_____

_____

_____

_____

What patterns or triggers lead you to make unconscious choices around food?

_____

_____

_____

_____

What would you like to change about your relationship with food so you can make more conscious choices?

_____

_____

_____

_____

What do you think would be the first step in making that change?

_____

_____

_____

_____

How would that positively impact your Best Energetic Self?

_____

_____

_____

_____

Attach your conscious choices to how you want to *feel*. If you're anything like me, you want to feel energized, motivated, comfortable, and confident. By learning to listen to your body and applying the other pillars—Thoughts, Mood, Digestion, Focus, and Energy Levels—you can make conscious choices that help you feel your best.

Conscious Choices With Food Deep Dive

Ask yourself: Is what I'm doing helping me feel how I want to? Does it support my Best Energetic Self? The answers to these questions and the flowchart at the top of this chapter will guide your decisions. Here's how I applied this in practice:

- I didn't want to feel tired anymore, so I chose to learn how to eat better.

- I didn't want to feel sluggish anymore, so I chose to learn how to relax without alcohol.
- I didn't want to feel gassy and bloated anymore, so I chose to figure out which foods were causing it.
- I wanted to feel comfortable in my body, so I chose to eat healthier.
- I wanted to feel energized, so I chose to eat enough protein.

Knowing is not the same as doing. Every decision I mentioned isn't a one-time choice—it's a daily commitment. I make these decisions to the best of my ability, and when I forget or don't have the capacity to follow through, I view it as a learning opportunity. Each time, I aim to do better and create an environment that makes it easier for me to succeed moving forward. How do we do this?

Setting up an environment for success simplifies the process of making conscious choices. Here are some tips to help you create a supportive eating environment:

- Keep your kitchen clean and equipped with tools and containers that make cooking easier.
- Create a pleasant space in your kitchen or dining room, such as adding decor or displaying fruit in bowls to make the space and fresh food feel inviting.
- Post notes on your refrigerator or set reminders for cooking and shopping.
- Move less supportive snacks to the back of the pantry.
- Prepare filling snacks or meals to have on hand from ingredients that support you.

As you've been learning about the *Energetic Eating Method* and the Triad of Health, remember that everything is connected. By creating an environment in which you can flourish, you'll notice the incredible impact it has on your Best Energetic Self. For instance, you might find that prioritizing nutrient-rich meals helps stabilize your mood and energy levels throughout the day, making it easier to stay productive and focused. Regular movement could improve your digestion and help you sleep more soundly at night. Mindfulness practices like journaling or meditation might reduce stress, allowing you to approach challenges with greater clarity and calm. These small, interconnected shifts can lead to a more vibrant, balanced, and empowered version of your Best Energetic Self.

Use the table or download it from the portal to reflect on changes you can make to set up an environment that supports your unique needs. Examples are provided to get you started.

PILLAR THAT COULD BE OUT OF BALANCE	SETTING UP MY ENVIRONMENT
Mood: Balance blood sugar, PM routines	*Put a journal next to my bed.*
Digestion: Explore your individual inflammatory foods, include foods that support digestion, and move more	*Make gluten-free avocado brownies for a treat.*
Focus: Include healthy fats, AM routines	*Prepare nuts on hand for a snack.*
Energy Levels: Include protein, midday breaks	*Put a sticky note reminder at my desk to take breaks every 50 minutes.*

PILLAR THAT COULD BE OUT OF BALANCE	SETTING UP MY ENVIRONMENT
Mood: Balance blood sugar, PM routines	
Digestion: Explore your individual inflammatory foods, include foods that support digestion, and move more	
Focus: Include healthy fats, AM Routines	
Energy Levels: Include protein, midday breaks	

Quick Look: Creating an Environment in Which You Can Flourish

- Reflect on what *creating an environment in which you can flourish* means to you.
- Revisit the pillars and consider which eating components and pillars might feel out of balance for you.
- Use the table provided or the printout in the book portal to evaluate what you need to set up an environment that supports you.

Now, we will explore the second affirmation of this chapter: *I cherish my relationships.*

THINK: *I cherish my relationships.*

How we connect with others and ourselves is one of the most profound parts of being human. It's no wonder we often prioritize the needs of others over our own. Women are especially taught to believe that keeping their kids and partners happy is the price of maintaining those relationships. We want them to be okay, but so often, we lose ourselves along the way.

What we forget is that we don't have to keep others happy for them to want to be around us. Positive energy and reciprocity naturally follow from showing up as your strongest Best Energetic Self. Taking care of yourself is an awe-inspiring act—it radiates outward, attracts others, and inspires them to care for themselves, too.

If we constantly bend over backward to appease others, we compromise our sense of self and well-being. This is where frustration and resentment creep in. We may feel paralyzed, unable to take action or start making choices for ourselves from a place of anger rather than health.

Fad diets perpetuate the belief that self-care must be separate from our relationships with the most important people in our lives. However, I believe that cherishing your relationships should be a part of your overall well-being. When you invest in continued acts of self-care, nourishment, and exercise, your relationships thrive. Your efforts to nurture yourself allow you to fully cherish those you love rather than feel resentment or seek escape.

When we're stuck in a diet mindset, it's easy to see our relationships as reasons to *not* take action—people and circumstances that don't "fit in." To overcome this, it's important to shift your mindset and recognize that your health isn't limited by others.

Use the provided space to write what the affirmation "I cherish my relationships" means to you.

I cherish my relationships.

Now that you've explored what it means to cherish your relationships, let's explore the "Live" portion of the triad as it relates to conscious choices.

LIVE: *Include People You Love*

My Story

I used to believe that my relationships with friends, family, and coworkers were separate from my health. Friendships were about indulging in baskets of french fries and margaritas, my role as a mom of a young child felt too overwhelming to think about caring for my own needs, and my work with colleagues always seemed to supersede exercise.

This, of course, like everything else, led me down the path of looking for quick fixes for health and weight loss. When life felt chaotic, diets became my go-to solution. I believed long-term healthy choices weren't possible with all my responsibilities, especially the ones to other people.

I remember being in the thick of parenting my 1-year-old. I wanted to squeeze in weight loss as quickly as possible because I didn't want to have to put my daughter and my full-time job on the backburner. I turned to a juice cleanse out of desperation. I convinced myself that something quick and easy was the only way to move the needle. For three days, I lived off frozen, pulpy juice bags I thawed each morning and swallowed down the chunks while ignoring my rumbling stomach and sleepless nights. By day four, I gave up. The remaining juice bags sat untouched in my freezer, crystallizing into frozen bricks. Like every other quick fix, this one failed. Like always, I thought my relationships took priority over my own health.

Here's the truth about what was going on for me: I held a limiting belief that taking care of myself long-term would *detract* from my relationships. I thought prioritizing my health could not have a symbiotic relationship with my personal life, but I was completely wrong.

When I stopped dieting and started listening to my body, my relationships actually flourished. My friends, family, and coworkers got interested in what I was doing. I invited my coworkers to run with me. My kids joined in on the workouts I would find online and eventually the ones I created for my clients, which instilled a love of exercise in them. My partner and I started weight training together. Even my friends noticed the changes in me—more patience, energy, and joy—and started making healthier choices themselves.

Cherishing my relationships no longer meant putting my long-term health last and the diet first. I discovered that nurturing myself strengthened my connections and helped me show up better for everyone in my life—including myself.

Health & Relationships Inventory

Let's take inventory of the connection between health and your relationships. You can write or use the space provided to reflect on the following questions:

When do you prioritize others' needs over your own?

_____

_____

_____

_____

How does this impact your physical and mental health?

_____

_____

_____

_____

What change would you like to make to incorporate health into your relationships?

_____

_____

_____

_____

What would be the first step in doing that?

_____

_____

_____

_____

How would that positively impact your Best Energetic Self?

_____

_____

_____

_____

Understanding the connections between your relationships and your health is an important first step. Now, let's explore the impact relationships have on health and well-being.

Health and Relationships Deep Dive

What if prioritizing your health didn't take away from your relationships but made them stronger?

Society often tells us that putting ourselves first is selfish, but the truth is that taking care of our health through movement, nourishing foods, and rest is one of the most selfless acts we can do. When we prioritize our well-being, we are more patient, present, and energized. Instead of running on empty, we give from a place of fullness, creating space for deeper, more meaningful connections with those we love.

We've all seen it—when we are stressed and overextended, it affects everything. We're quicker to snap at our kids, less patient with our partners, and even our friendships can start to feel like obligations. But when we take care of our health—whether it's through exercise, nourishing food, or simply taking a break—we're able to bring a different energy into those relationships. We become role models for the people around us. Our children start to see what it looks like to value health and well-being, and they begin to mirror those choices. Our partners feel the difference in our energy, and the connection deepens. Our friends are inspired to make healthier choices when they see our changes. We become a source of strength and inspiration. Taking care of our health is an act of love—not just for ourselves but for everyone who depends on us. It's a powerful cycle where our well-being feeds the well-being of our relationships, and our relationships, in turn, support our health.

Quick Look: Health and Relationships

- Reflect on what it means to you to cherish your relationships alongside your health and well-being.
- Look for opportunities to invite friends, family, and colleagues into your health journey.
- Follow through with your actions even when you feel a responsibility to others, and see what happens!

The Power of Conscious Choices with Relationships and Your Environment

Because I make conscious choices for my health, I now honor my body and the way I want to feel each day. Every decision is rooted in becoming my Best Energetic Self. I know that when I choose what makes me feel good, I carry it through all aspects of my life. I surround myself with nourishing foods, ensuring I eat well consistently. I've created a dedicated space at home for working out in my basement and lay my workout clothes out at night so I never have an excuse to skip my movement for the day. My bedside table holds a journal and crossword puzzles, helping me ease into restful sleep. These choices have not only been a part of my transformation but also impacted the people I love. My younger daughter joins my workouts and now creates her own exercise routines. My older daughter has learned how to tailor her meals to her gluten-sensitive needs. Giving up alcohol has inspired many of my friends to drink less or do the same.

Every day, I encourage my clients to make conscious choices for their health and well-being. This is what makes health sustainable—it's not about chasing a number on a scale but about living a life filled with energy and balance. When we approach health as a series of intentional choices, we create a lasting foundation that supports not only our physical bodies, but our overall quality of life.

Use the *Energetic Eating Journal* exercise to explore how making conscious choices from this chapter can help you. Prompts are given to help you if you feel stuck.

Date: _____

MIT(s): *What is the most important thing that you learned from this chapter?*		
How I Think:	How I Eat:	How I Live:
What is a positive thought or affirmation that you would like to take with you?	*When you think about supporting yourself nutritionally, what could that look like now?*	*When you think about supporting yourself through lifestyle choices, what could that look like now?*

| Breakfast: |
| How did you feel? |

| Lunch: |
| How did you feel? |

| Dinner: |
| How did you feel? |

| Snack 1: | Snack 2: |
| How did you feel? | How did you feel? |

| Liquids: |
| How did you feel? |

Reflection: *How are you feeling today? What conscious choices did you make with your thoughts, eating, and lifestyle?*

PART III:
BRINGING IT ALL TOGETHER

CHAPTER 10

PRIORITIZING YOUR HEALTH BRINGS JOY AND BALANCE

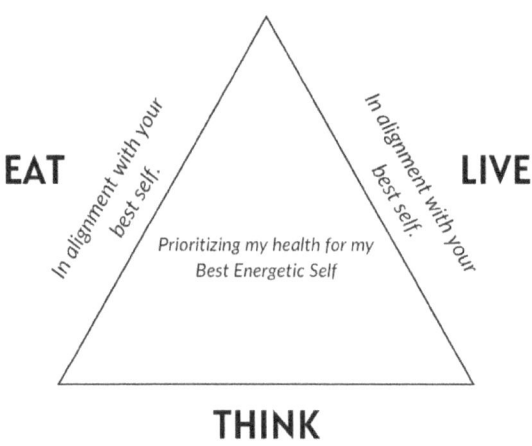

In this chapter, through The Think, Eat, Live Triad, we'll examine the final affirmation, "Prioritizing my health brings joy and balance," for your Best Energetic Self.

Overview

We've now completed our journey through all Six Pillars of Energetic Eating! It's time to focus on putting everything you've learned into action by making your health a top priority.

We often think about health as something we need to get around to, something we'll prioritize once life slows down. But what if we connected our health to the bigger vision we have for ourselves? What if our Best Energetic Self—the version of us that we dream about, the one that shows up fully in every area of life—is actually a product of the healthy choices we make?

That's what *Energetic Eating* has been about. It's an installation of habits and tools, a way to think, eat, and live that goes beyond the surface and deep into the energetic body. You might have believed that weight loss was the key, that once the pounds were gone, you'd finally show up as the person you've always wanted to be. My hope is that you've realized that the weight is secondary to the transformation happening deep within.

The habits you build will change how you see food and how you see your life. No longer will you force yourself into a rigid mold of dieting, hating your body, and trying to fix it without understanding the underlying causes. That version of you—the one that punished herself and fought against her body—will be history. Now you will align with your vision. You'll embrace the idea that health is about loving your life enough to make the changes necessary, using the pillars you've learned. You'll do the inner work. You'll clear your energy and move forward, ready to build on these habits for years to come.

What we've learned together is that practicing *Energetic Eating*—thinking, eating, and living day in and day out for your Best Energetic Self—isn't just something we do temporarily. It's the foundation for our lives. It's what we must cultivate so deeply that it becomes second nature, so ingrained that it feels harder *not* to do it.

Prioritizing Health Reflection

Rate each of the following on a scale of 1–5, with 1 meaning "never," 3 meaning "sometimes," and 5 meaning "always." Consider these questions in relation to the past six months.

- Do you make your health the last thing on your to-do list?
- Do you believe you can't prioritize your health ahead of other responsibilities?
- Do you find yourself feeling overwhelmed by the thought of daily healthy choices?
- Do you ever avoid prioritizing your health because you're afraid what you try won't work or be good enough?
- Do you view prioritizing your health as a luxury rather than a necessity?

Total: ___ out of 25

If you scored 15 or higher, the suggestions in this chapter will be especially helpful for you to explore and implement.

THINK: *Prioritizing my health brings joy and balance.*

When we make our health a priority, we are fueling the vessel that we use to navigate the world as powerfully as possible. However, we have been taught that our health is something we need to carve out time for after we finish everything else and that taking care of ourselves is separate and more difficult than anything else in our lives. But prioritizing our health, while challenging at times, actually makes everything else easier and makes it possible for our bodies to no longer be distractions, ultimately leading to joy, balance, and any truth we are seeking as our Best Energetic Selves.

Each day presents an opportunity for us to focus on the most important drivers of our health—the thoughts, foods, and behaviors that help us meet our needs. *That* is health. It's not just exercising, eating right, or sleeping well—it is using those things to be who we truly want to be.

Our bodies, our emotions, and our lives do not exist in a vacuum. There are other people, demands, needs, shoulds, wants, and desires. We will occasionally choose those things over our health. It is totally normal and natural to play with boundaries, test the waters, and negotiate your priorities. It is normal to feel tired sometimes. It's normal to feel like you don't want to do something, to go into avoidance, or for old habits to rear their heads. Change won't be overnight, and that's okay. It's a journey. Prioritizing your Best Energetic Self may have ups and downs, but I promise it will bring you joy and balance.

To overcome the limitations of your thoughts and personal history with dieting, use the space provided to reflect on what this affirmation means to you.

Prioritizing my health brings joy and balance.

Now that you understand how prioritizing your health brings joy and balance, let's see how you can connect your health with your best self.

Connecting Your Health to Your Best Energetic Self

As humans, we crave challenges. We say we want things to be easy, but ease alone isn't fulfilling. And because prioritizing health isn't easy (at least not at first), there will likely come a point when the rebellious part of you wants to throw in the towel. You might feel restless or bored, like you're done with this journey. That voice will whisper, *"Why can't I just do what I want?"*

The danger is that we often mistake that voice as permission to return to old habits. We think, *"I'm sick of this,"* and drift back to what's familiar. But what if, instead of letting that urge pull us backward, we used it as a signal to rise? What if, in those moments, we looked to our Best Energetic Self as inspiration—not to give up, but to step up?

Before you continue, reread your Best Energetic Self from Chapter 3. Close your eyes and imagine what it feels like to achieve that vision. Set a two-minute timer to connect with that part of yourself using all your senses. What do you feel, see, smell, hear, and taste? Put yourself in the places and with the people that support you.

In the table below or in a journal, write down ideas for how to align your conscious choices with your Best Energetic Self based on the tools and habits you've learned in this book.

Below, you'll see my example, followed by a blank template. Feel free to print it out for yourself using the resource in the book portal.

	How I Think	How I Eat	How I Live
My Best Self: Successful entrepreneur, author, and speaker Loving and committed Mom and partner Strong, fit, and energized, without body distractions	Tape the affirmations on my mirror, so I speak kindly to myself Write a gratitude list every day, so I release negativity	Fresh-cut vegetables are always available, and fruit is in a bowl on my counter top so I remember health is a priority Put the tea next to the coffee to remind myself to relax instead of always be on the go Print out my meal plan for the week and put it on the fridge so I am prepared	Keep an AM/PM journal next to my bed to release stress and welcome in the day Put a sticky note on my computer reminding me to move, shift, or burpee every 20 minutes so I have work/life balance Place a yoga mat in the TV room for early morning stretching and AM routine

Quick Look: Prioritizing Your Health for Your Best Energetic Self

- Reflect on what it means to "Prioritize your health."
- Reread your Best Energetic Self
- Consider what components from the Triad of Health are most important to you right now to be successful

Your Continued Energetic Eating Journaling Process

At the end of every pillar, you have had a chance to complete a journaling exercise to help you integrate what you've learned. Keeping a journal is an effective way to not just dump your thoughts and prepare for your day, but also to keep yourself on track. I ebb and flow with my *Energetic Eating* journal practice. Sometimes, I do it every evening and every morning, and sometimes I do it only when I need it, such as returning from vacation or holidays when I can feel vulnerable about my body and detached from *Energetic Eating*.

I do not write down my food unless I feel like one of the pillars is out of balance. When a pillar is out of balance, journaling my food helps me slow down and feel more present with my eating habits so that I can identify what might be triggering me to feel badly in my body. When that is the case, I will journal exactly how I have taught you. I write down my most important things and then how I will think, eat, and live, followed by what I will eat that day. I hold myself accountable and recognize the need for change. I will hear myself say, "Oh yeah! I am feeling tired. It's time to balance my blood sugar using what I know about mood," or, "Oh right! I am going to grab some nuts instead of a snack bar because I am feeling a lack of focus."

The point is that I get to decide how I want to show up based on how I feel and what will support my Best Energetic Self that day. Below is an example of your daily journal entry sheet. You can draw it in a journal or download more in the book portal.

MIT(s): *What is the most important thing you'd like to focus on from your Best Energetic Self?*

How I Think:	How I Eat:	How I Live:
What is a positive thought or affirmation that you would like to take with you?	*When you think about supporting yourself nutritionally, what could that look like now?*	*When you think about supporting yourself through lifestyle choices, what could that look like now?*

Breakfast: How did you feel?
Lunch: How did you feel?
Dinner: How did you feel?

Snack 1: How did you feel?	Snack 2: How did you feel?

Liquids: How did you feel?
Reflection: *How are you feeling today? How has making these shifts positively influenced your Best Energetic Self?*

CHAPTER 11

LOOKING BACK, LOOKING FORWARD

Looking Back

I want you to write a letter to your past self.

To start, go back to the core memories you wrote down in the Thoughts Pillar. I want you to write to *her* about her experience with dieting, weight loss, and weight gain. I want you to get into her mind—the things she was thinking about and the things she was worrying about.

Using the tools and journal entries from this book, you are going to tell your past self what she needs to do to address current challenges or the ones coming in the years that follow. You are going to look at her, with compassion and grace, and give her the courage and the advice that you didn't have before. You are going to make who you are today be the powerful all-knowing. You're the one not just with the wisdom of experience but with the strength to change.

What are the important things for her to think about and focus on? What does she need to know about how to think, eat, and live to take care of herself? What does she need to know about the Six Pillars of Health? Tell her how far you've come and all you know. Because today, in this moment you are more than just the past—you are capable of molding and framing your future. After this exercise, you will complete another Best Energetic Self.

Write this letter to yourself in a journal, on a sheet of paper, or in the provided space.

Looking Forward to Your Best Energetic Self

You are going to write your Best Energetic Self again. You might find now that you are able to go more richly and deeply into your vision after everything you have learned. What haven't you fully committed to yet from the Best Energetic Self that you envisioned in Chapter 3? What can you add to your Best Energetic Self that you didn't include before?

Your Best Energetic Self

Imagine I could wave a magic wand and instantly grant you your ideal health. Picture yourself six months from now—feeling, vibrant, energetic, confident, and completely at ease in your body. How do you feel? What does your daily routine look like? What choices are you making? Use the three sections provided to explore different facets of your transformation.

Career, work, service, finances:

Relationships, home, travel, intimacy:

Health, spirituality, home-cooking, exercise:

This is your chance to reclaim your health with small, manageable steps—an opportunity to break free from the cycle of quick fixes and create lasting, sustainable changes so you no longer have to carry the burden of weight fluctuations and fad dieting.

Don't stop reaching for your Best Energetic Self. Shift your thoughts into energy that uplifts you, choose foods that truly nourish you, and take actions for a lifestyle that fully supports you. Stay attuned to your body's signals—they're always guiding you. Listen for what supports your thoughts, mood, digestion, focus, energy levels, and conscious choices, and honor them with intention.

Remember—*Energetic Eating* isn't just about food. What you've practiced here can extend into every part of your life. You can apply these tools to how you work, how you connect with people, how you honor your well-being, and even how you pursue your passions. Every conscious choice is an opportunity to create alignment, balance, and fulfillment—not just on your plate, but in your entire life.

It's been such a privilege to walk this *Energetic Eating* journey with you. The work you've done is powerful, and I'm excited to see where it takes you next—not just for you, but for every woman daring to redefine health on her own terms. Keep showing up for yourself—you deserve it.

Now that you've heard my story and seen the incredible shifts that *Energetic Eating* has created in my life and the lives of my clients, it's time to meet more inspiring women who began their journeys seeking weight loss but discovered something far greater—empowerment. These women have generously shared their stories to inspire you, remind you of what's possible, and encourage you to stay courageous and committed to becoming your Best Energetic Self through *Energetic Eating*.

CHAPTER 12

ENERGETIC EATING METHOD CLIENT SUCCESS STORIES

Stephanie: The power of attuning to your body's needs

Stephanie came to me at a pivotal moment in her life. As a woman in her 40s and a mother of two, she had heard all the common refrains: "Your body won't change now that you've had kids" or "It's too late to make a difference." But what stood out about Stephanie was her refusal to accept those limiting beliefs. Through the *Energetic Eating Method*, she began to truly understand the power of attuning herself to her body's needs rather than living by rigid food rules. For her, it wasn't about deprivation or dieting anymore—it was about freedom and balance.

She described how, in the past, she would have obsessed and overcompensated for holiday meals, constantly worrying about her next diet or the repercussions of a few indulgent moments. "I remember feeling exactly like that, and it feels really good being free from it now," she said, reflecting on how her mindset had shifted. This sense of freedom extended into her daily life. Stephanie realized she could enjoy foods that once seemed "off-limits" and without guilt, as long as she was in tune with how they made her feel. "If I'm at a movie and feel like having an ice cream, I'm pretty sure I'm going to have one. It's fine because I know my body and how to balance it out."

What struck me most about Stephanie's journey was her deep understanding of balance—both in food and life. She shared a story about meeting a friend for lunch, where a simple sandwich left her feeling sluggish. But instead of spiraling into guilt, she accepted the moment for what it was and moved on. "I knew I needed a nap, but it was fine. I just listened to my body." That type of self-awareness is at the heart of the *Energetic Eating Method*—knowing when something feels off but also knowing how to course-correct without judgment.

Of course, the occasional indulgence happens, and Stephanie admitted to having moments where she might drink a little too much or eat more than she planned. But she learned to avoid the shame spiral. "It's hard to avoid those negative thoughts, but I remind myself it will pass," she explained. Instead of staying stuck, she leaned on the practices she knew would pull her back—exercise, hydration, rest. These were her tools for regaining balance. "I know what works for me," she said, "and if I get back into my routine, I know I'll feel fine again."

Stephanie's journey wasn't just about making healthier food choices; it was about redefining her relationship with herself. When asked what drives her today, she didn't mention weight loss or fitting into a certain size. Instead, she talked about the things that truly matter to her—learning flamenco in Spain, speaking Spanish, and showing her children what it means to live a fulfilling life. "I'm here in Spain because I fought for it really hard. I want to experience life, and I wake up every day wanting to do my best," she shared.

Stephanie's transformation was less about her body and more about becoming her best energetic self.

Her message to anyone considering the *Energetic Eating Method*? "It will reconcile you with yourself. By the end of this, you will love yourself so much more. And that's a gift anyone should give themselves."

Emma: Breaking free from the diet trap

Emma's initial goal upon entering the program was to feel confident enough to take photos with her children, something she had avoided for years. She wanted to cultivate energy not just for her kids but also to reconnect with herself outside of motherhood. Reflecting on her experience, Emma recalled how becoming a mother during the COVID-19 pandemic shifted her routine. Living in New York, she was active and consumed healthy meals effortlessly. However, after giving birth and transitioning to a more confined lifestyle, her health took a backseat. The ease of ordering takeout replaced the healthy habits she had built, leading to weight gain and a sense of frustration with her self-image.

Emma articulated a profound realization: there never seemed to be a "right time" to prioritize her health amidst the challenges of motherhood and a pandemic. This cycle of postponing self-care took a toll not only on her physical health but also on her self-esteem and energy levels. Recognizing this pattern was a pivotal moment in her journey, one that led her to the *Energetic Eating Method*.

In her previous attempts to manage her weight, Emma found herself trapped in the restrictive mindset of calorie counting and exercise tracking, which ultimately drained the joy from her meals and social experiences. She recounted how these habits, while effective in the short term, left her feeling disconnected from nourishing her body. With the *Energetic Eating Method*, Emma discovered a different approach—one focused on enjoying food that genuinely made her feel good.

Emma now embraces a philosophy of nourishment rather than restriction. She prioritizes protein and aims for a diverse array of vegetables, making a mental note of her progress without the confines of tracking calories. One of the most liberating aspects for her has been the absence of "bad" foods; she no longer views certain foods as forbidden. Instead, she approaches meals with a mindset of balance and enjoyment.

Emma's transformation was not just physical; it was mental and emotional. She shifted from an all-or-nothing mindset to one of resilience and self-compassion. Even when facing setbacks, like illness in her family, she no longer succumbs to old habits. Instead, she stays engaged with the program, learning and growing, affirming that life's challenges are opportunities for practice rather than reasons to give up. After the program, Emma suggests how other women can do the same:

1. Focus on Nourishment: Prioritize protein and a colorful array of vegetables to fuel your body effectively.

2. Reframe Your Mindset: Understand that no foods are inherently bad. Allow yourself the freedom to enjoy a variety of foods while still aiming for balanced nutrition.

3. Practice Self-Compassion: Embrace the journey with flexibility. Recognize that setbacks are part of the process, and continue learning and growing without judgment.

Emma's story is a powerful reminder that health is a personal journey. By redefining her relationship with food and herself, she not only took charge of her health but also taught her children the value of balance and self-love.

Shar: Finding balance in body and mind

Shar, a busy midwife, mom, and graduate student, came to the *Energetic Eating Method* feeling overwhelmed and burdened by the extra weight she had gained during menopause. Balancing the demands of her career, motherhood, and school, she had little time to focus on her own health. The constant juggling act left her feeling stuck, both physically and emotionally. After years of trying various diets that never seemed to work, Shar was searching for something different—something that would help her find balance in her body and life.

"The promise of a different way to balance my life and body resonated with me," Shar shared when asked why she chose this method over others. The *Energetic Eating Method* wasn't just another quick fix; it offered her a holistic approach that addressed both her physical health and her emotional well-being. The weight came off, but perhaps even more important was the inner shift. Shar learned how to love herself along the way, discovering the power of self-compassion amidst her busy life.

Reflecting on where she'd be if she hadn't embraced the *Energetic Eating Method*, Shar shared, "I would still be sitting on the couch." Instead, her life has transformed. She now attends Pilates three times a week, listens to her body when it comes to eating—cutting back on gluten, which has caused joint pain and overeating—and limits her alcohol intake. Each day, she reminds herself that years of yo-yo dieting had kept her stuck in a cycle of calorie counting and obsessively tracking points. Now free from that mental burden, Shar feels the weight of that alternative life slipping away. For her, the *Energetic Eating Method* has been more than just a weight-loss journey; it has been a profound transformation, helping her navigate menopause and life's demands with renewed energy and deepened self-love.

Jill D: From Restriction to Conscious Choices

Jill started her journey with *Energetic Eating* believing she was already eating "healthy foods." However, her understanding of health changed when she realized the importance of checking ingredients and understanding how food affects the body. She learned that labels can be misleading—products marketed as "healthy" aren't always beneficial for her body. This shift empowered Jill to make more informed choices and embrace conscious eating.

One of Jill's biggest transformations was moving away from restrictive diets. She had tried countless diets that labeled foods as "good" or "bad," leaving her feeling resentful and limited. With *Energetic Eating*, she now makes choices based on what feels good for her body, not what she's allowed or not allowed to eat. She's even been able to reframe how she approaches food with her children, teaching them that healthy eating is about choice, not restriction.

Jill describes how her new mindset allows her to enjoy food without guilt. For example, when dining out with friends, she can savor a bite of dessert and put the spoon down without feeling the need to overindulge. In the past, this type of situation might have led to overeating or feeling guilt and regret the next day. Now, she feels more balanced, knowing she can make healthy choices again with the next meal.

Jill also emphasizes the power of community in her success. She believes it's incredibly difficult to make these changes alone. The support and encouragement she's received have been key to maintaining her mindset shift, helping her see food through a positive, loving lens rather than a critical one.

For Jill, *Energetic Eating* is not just about physical transformation but also mental freedom. She no longer feels the pressure of constantly worrying about her food intake or body size. Instead, her focus has shifted to being present with her family and feeling energized in her daily life. The ability to make conscious, empowering choices has given her peace of mind and a deeper connection with her body.

Jill M: Shifting strategy from weight-based to health-based

Jill's journey with the *Energetic Eating Method* is a powerful example of how shifting from a weight-focused approach to a holistic view of health can transform not only one's relationship with food but also their overall well-being. When Jill started the program, she shared that her previous experience with dieting had been rooted in restriction and a constant obsession with the number on the scale. "All I've done in the past is restrict food, exercise for weight loss, get on the scale, become frustrated, and rinse and repeat," she explained. The focus was never on health but rather on conforming to societal standards of what a 'thin woman' should look like.

Through the *Energetic Eating Method*, Jill learned to approach food and exercise from a new perspective focused on health and well-being rather than just aesthetics. She began to understand the importance of nourishing her body and moving in ways that support her mental and physical health. This shift helped her release the rigid mindset of dieting and embrace a more balanced and conscious approach to eating.

An example of this shift came when Jill visited her son for a parents' weekend at college. Faced with a less-than-healthy breakfast menu, she made a conscious choice. "Instead of saying, 'I'm just writing this weekend off and eating whatever I want,' I looked at the menu and decided to have an omelet with cheese and one piece of toast instead of the four slices they gave me. I knew that would fill me up and wouldn't give me a bellyache." This decision reflected her newfound ability to balance enjoyment with her physical well-being.

Jill also spoke about how the program helped her avoid guilt around food. In moments when she might have made a less optimal choice, she learned to practice self-compassion.

"When I make the less healthy choice, it feeds into the old story. So, when I'm successful, it's self-compassion. I made the best choice for me in that circumstance, and even if I didn't, it's not as big of a deal as my brain's making it out to be." Instead of feeling trapped in guilt, she began to view her body's reactions as information, using a detective mindset to understand what felt good and what didn't.

The program's unique approach to empowerment also stood out to Jill. She shared a story about dining at a burger place with her family. Knowing the food would make her feel unwell, she chose to bring her own salad from a nearby restaurant. "I gave myself permission to go get myself a salad and bring it over. It wasn't worth it to me to eat a burger because I knew I was going to get a stomach ache." This empowered choice was a departure from the past when she might have just gone along with everyone else.

Jill's advice to those starting the program is simple but profound: "Lean into the program. It's a wholly different way of approaching physical and emotional health, and for people in my generation [40-something women], it's a new muscle to build. But when you trust your body and listen to it, the results are lasting and go beyond the scale."

Her success story is a testament to the transformative power of trusting oneself, practicing self-compassion, and making conscious choices that honor the body. Through the *Energetic Eating Method,* Jill has found a sustainable and empowering path to health.

Brenda: Transforming relationships with food and self-love

Brenda and I delved deep into how the *Energetic Eating Method* approach has profoundly impacted her relationship with food and overall well-being. Her journey began with a familiar struggle—food was a source of confusion and contention. But through the *Energetic Eating Method*, that relationship shifted dramatically.

Brenda described how she now views food as a way to nourish and energize her body, aligning it with her personal goals. "Before, I followed someone else's diet or plan, and it just didn't fit me. But now I know what works for me, and that makes all the difference," she explained. This shift highlights the power of conscious choices—food no longer carries value judgments. Instead, it's about understanding how it fuels your unique body and what feels right for you.

One of the most significant shifts Brenda experienced was moving away from guilt. She shared how this was a game-changer: "When I make a choice that may not be ideal, I don't spiral into guilt. I look at it as information, just one moment in time, not a failure." This mindset—shifting from guilt to curiosity—allowed her to maintain momentum on her journey. "You can just keep going. I didn't miss a step or fail. I learned something, and now I know more."

For Brenda, conscious choices became synonymous with self-love. By learning what foods work best for her and understanding how to fuel her body in alignment with her goals, she began to embody self-compassion. "It's like I'm in the driver's seat now. I choose what my body needs, not some restrictive diet plan," she reflected.

One practice Brenda embraced was journaling, both in the form of food logs and setting daily intentions. These exercises helped her stay mindful and connected to her goals, while the community aspect of the program provided accountability. "I thought I had to do it all on my own, but the group support made such a difference."

Brenda also emphasized the importance of aligning her personal goals—whether related to family, work, or life passions—with her health choices. "I realized my goals weren't about body type or weight number. They were about having the energy to be there for my children and achieve what I want in life," she said. This revelation helped her move beyond temporary fixes and focus on long-term health and vitality.

When asked about the one mindset shift that made the most impact, Brenda mentioned her favorite affirmation: "I always know the next right action." She found that taking one small, manageable step at a time allowed her to avoid feeling overwhelmed and stay focused on her journey. This approach not only fostered progress but also cultivated a deeper sense of self-love.

ACKNOWLEDGMENTS

This book would not have been possible without the incredible support, guidance, and inspiration of so many people in my life.

First, to my clients—you are the heart and soul of this work. Your courage to show up for yourselves and take ownership of your health inspires me every single day. Thank you for trusting me with your journeys, for teaching me more than I could ever learn alone, and for being a part of a community that uplifts and empowers women everywhere. This book is as much yours as it is mine. The years we have spent together have profoundly shaped my ideas, deepened my understanding of what true health looks like, and kept me motivated to complete this book.

To my partner, who not only stood by me during this process but also rolled up her sleeves to help me edit and revise this book—you are my biggest supporter. Your thoughtful feedback, tireless encouragement, and belief in this project gave me the confidence to keep going, even when it felt overwhelming.

To my family—thank you for your unconditional love and belief in me and my larger-than-life visions. You have been a source of strength and grounding for me. To my friends, who have been my sounding boards and cheerleaders, and to the women who have come before us, paving the way for a more inclusive, empowering, and supportive world for health and wellness, thank you.

To my past self—thank you for never giving up, even in the face of addiction, weight struggles, and self-doubt. The lessons from those years have given me the empathy, compassion, and determination to create this work for others.

And to you, the reader—thank you for picking up this book and embarking on this journey. I see you, and I believe in you. Together, we are creating a ripple effect of change that will make the world a better, healthier place for generations of women to come.

With gratitude,
Helen

ABOUT THE AUTHOR

Helen is the Founder of the *Energetic Eating Method* and CEO of Cultivate Health Coaching, helping women reclaim their health with an empowering, holistic approach to nutrition and lifestyle. She guides women to reconnect with their bodies, shift limiting beliefs, and break free from the cycles of fad dieting—so they can create lasting, sustainable well-being.

With a communications, media, and education background, Helen's academic journey reflects her deep commitment to transformation. She holds degrees from Ohio University, The New School, and Bank Street College of Education, along with specialized training in health and wellness from the Institute for Integrative Nutrition, Optimize Life Coaching, The Kinesiology Institute, and other leading programs.

Blending personal experience, extensive education, and years of coaching, Helen believes health is not a number on a scale—it's a powerful, dynamic balance of mind, body, and self. Her approach combines science-backed strategies with subtle energy work, creating profound, lasting transformation for the women she serves. As an active community member and a mom to two children who inspire her daily, she understands firsthand the importance of creating a healthy, balanced life that supports personal well-being and those we love.

www.ingramcontent.com/pod-product-compliance
Lightning Source LLC
Chambersburg PA
CBHW020534030426
42337CB00013B/853